Essential Oils:

100% Organic Recipes For Healing Salves, Deodorants, Shampoos and Body Washes

Table of Contents

Introduction

Essential oils are extracted from plants. There are several purposes of using essential oils. It is good to be proactive about talking to qualified individuals and doing research in finding out the facts.

There are primarily three ways to enter essential oils in your body. You can inhale them, apply them on your body or ingest them. The selected application method mainly depends on two factors, the chosen oil, and the desired effects.

Essential oils are used for treating acne, aches, and anxiety from ancient Egypt and China to present day. Each plant has a distinctive smell. Every scent has unique healing qualities.

Essential oils can do wonders for your hair and skin. Some of the essential oils improve your scalp while others do wonders on your hair. Aromatherapy is an effective remedy for hormone imbalance and anxiety. Many of the hurdles to losing weight are psychological, such depressed moods, and emotional eating. Aromatherapy can be the missing piece in your struggle to lose weight. They also play a useful role in relieving stress and anxiety.

Chapter 1 – All About Essential Oils

Essential oil is the essence of the plant; this essence of the plant is the part which contains the fragrance. Plants produce chemicals that attract pollinators as well as chemicals that repel predators. These chemicals are for the most part, the plants essential oil. Essential oil is not always an oil per se, it's insolubility in water is one of the reasons it is called oil, these oils are concentrated hydrophobic liquids.

The oil is extracted from the plant in several ways; distillation, cold press, solvent extraction, absolute oil extraction, and expression. The oils are used to flavor foods, scent soap and cleaning fluids, incense, cosmetics, perfumes, and for medicinal purposes. It is important to do a little research when looking to purchase essential oils; as with all products, some oils are better than others.

Essential oils are volatile; volatility is a term used in physics to explain a compounds tendency to evaporate. So, essential oils evaporate. Using essential oils at home is safe as long as the user understands the properties. Essential oil can act as a solvent and remove nail polish and even eat through a foam cup. Never touch your eyes or any other surface if you have essential oil on your fingers or hand. Use a dropper when working with essential oils.

There are many ways to use and work with essential oils. The concentrate itself is very rarely used alone, it is mixed with other oils or water. The oils used with essential oils are called carrier oils. A carrier oil is unscented; this makes it perfect for adding essential oils for fragrance. Although water and essential oil do not mix well, when water is used, the resulting mixture must be shaken before use to disperse the oil to create a blend.

This is a list of commonly used essential oils, this is only for informative use only, it is not complete guide for use.

Commonly Used Essential Oils:

Anise Oil – Smells like licorice and is used medicinally. It has decongestant properties, enhances libido, works as a stimulant and is fragrant and frequently used in food processing and flavoring

Bay Oil – Used in perfumes and aromatherapy. It is an analgesic, antiseptic, it has a spicy aroma and it has sedative properties

Bergamot Oil – Used in perfumes and aromatherapy. This oil has deodorant properties disinfectant, is an anti-depressant and it supports a healthy digestive system

Chamomile Oil – Used for medicinal properties, both Roman and German are used, German has a higher anti-inflammatory compound. It has antiseptic properties, aids in digestion, and works to relieve depression. This also has sedative properties to help induce a restful sleep

Cedarwood Oil – Used for its fragrance. Cedarwood has sedative properties, it is an antiseptic and anti-inflammatory

Cinnamon Oil – Used for flavor and medicinal properties. It increases libido, enhances the immune system, increases circulation and relieves depression

Clove Oil – Used as a topical anesthetic for dental pain. It relives coughs, and helps with respiratory issues

Eucalyptus Oil – Medicinal use for coughs and colds, has germicidal properties and is a good decongestant

Jasmine Oil – Used for its fragrance. It has sedative properties, relieves stress and anxiety, raises libido and is an aphrodisiac

Lavender Oil – Used for fragrance and medicinal properties. It is antiseptic, relaxes nerves and has sedative properties

Lemon Oil – Used medicinally, as an antiseptic, and in cosmetics. It is stimulating and helps cognitive function and aids in digestion

Marjoram Oil – Medicinal uses and for aromatherapy. This oil has analgesic properties, is a sedative, and it has antiviral properties

Patchouli Oil – For perfumes, medicinal, and aromatherapy. It is an aphrodisiac, antidepressant and it supports a peaceful feeling

Peppermint Oil – Medicinal uses and aromatherapy. It is a stimulant, it improves focus and concentration, and has anti-inflammatory properties

Rose Oil – Used for its fragrance. It is an aphrodisiac, improves depression and raises the libido

Rosemary Oil – Used medicinally and in aromatherapy. It relieves headaches, improves clarity, learning, and memory

Sandalwood Oil – Used for its fragrance. It improves memory and clarity, promotes a calm feeling, is anti-inflammatory and antiseptic

Tea Tree Oil – Used for medicinal properties. Improves earaches, bad breath, and cold sores. It supports a healthy respiratory system

Ylang-Ylang Oil – Used for medicinal properties and in aromatherapy. Supports heart health, and improves mood. It is an aphrodisiac and improves libido

This list is just an example of the essential oils commonly used. These oils are a good starting place for learning about the uses of essential oils. If you plan to use essential oils for medicinal purposes you will need a comprehensive list with detailed information on the medicinal properties of essential oil.

Essential oil is the ingredient in homemade body spray that adds fragrance. The more you learn about essential oils the more freedom you will have in creating your own scents. The recipes in this book will provide you with a starting point, you can learn to personalize your fragrances when you become familiar with essential oils and the varying scents and properties.

Some essential oil can be caustic to skin; it can cause a rash or sensitivity. Mugwart is an essential oil that has been used for centuries but today it is understood as a neurotoxin. It is important to know about the oil you want to use, there are many book available that focus on essential oil and its properties.

This essential oil chart shows what the plant looks like, and gives information on the properties of the oil. This is only an example, but it shows some of the many healthful benefits derived from essential oils.

Chapter 2. Amazing Recipes for All Occasions

Basic Body Spray

8 oz. of distilled water (distilled water is boiled and the steam is collected in a clean container; this removes most impurities)

1 Table Spoon of witch hazel (witch hazel takes the place of alcohol, it is gentler and has skin soothing properties)

20 -30 drops of essential oil

A spray pump bottle that will hold 8 oz. or more

Directions:

In the spray bottle, mix the distilled water with the witch hazel, and then add the essential oil/oils. Make sure the pump is on tight and shake the mixture well. Essential oil does not blend with water, it eventually separates, you will have to shake your spray before each use.

The following are recipes for body sprays, each recipe has different parts of essential oil added to the basic body spray:

Uplifting and Energizing: 5 drops of lavender oil and 15 drops of grapefruit oil.

Cozy and Romantic: 10 drops of cinnamon leaf oil and 15 drops of sweet orange oil.

Concentration and Focus: 5 drops of rosemary oil, 10 drops of peppermint oil, and 10 drops of patchouli oil.

Romantic Evening: 15 drops of rose oil and 10 drops of ylang-ylang.

Sweet Dreams: 15 drops of lavender oil and 10 drops of roman chamomile oil.

Winter Wonderland: 5 drops of vanilla oil (vanilla extract), 10 drops of cinnamon leaf oil, and 10 drops of sweet orange oil.

Banish the Blues: 10 drops of lavender oil and 10 drops of lemon oil.

Final Exam Focus Potion: 5 drops of lemon oil, 5 drops of black pepper oil, and 10 drops of peppermint oil.

Confident and Calm: 10 drops of rosemary oil, 5 drops of grapefruit oil, and 10 drops of geranium oil.

Peaceful Joy: 10 drops of frankincense oil and 10 drops of geranium oil.

Daydream Bliss: 10 drops of tea tree oil, 10 drops of lavender oil, and 5 drops of geranium oil.

Now that you have an idea of how much to use you should experiment with combinations of your own. You can begin by changing the amounts in these recipes to see what affect it has on the scent. Everyone is different, you may prefer more lavender and less tea tree in the Daydream Bliss recipe, so play around with the scents and amounts.

This is a list of essential oil and the effects they have on emotions and moods:

Sleep	Romance	Relaxation	Rejuvenation	Stress Relief	Happiness
Lavender	Rose	Lavender	Wintergreen	Geranium	Lemon
Roman Chamomile	Ylang-Ylang	Frankincense	Basil	Rose	Orange
Clary Sage	Neroli	Cedarwood	Wild Orange	Bergamot	Rose
Bergamot	Jasmine	German Chamomile	Lemon	Marjoram	Ginger
Frankincense	Sandalwood	Jasmine	Peppermint	Chamomile	Clove
Ylang-Ylang	Patchouli	Geranium	Cinnamon	Vetiver	Jasmine
Marjoram	Amyris	Frankincense	Rosemary	Rosewood	Geranium

Vanilla Lavender Perfume

Ingredients:

- 20 drops of lavender essential oil

- 15 drops of vanilla extract

- two vanilla beans

- once cup lavender flowers, dried

- two tablespoons of vegetable glycerin

- half a cup of witch hazel

Directions:

Using a sharp knife slice the vanilla beans open. Put the beans and the flowers in a large glass jar with a lid. Pour the witch hazel into the jar and secure the lid. Let this mix infuse for the next two weeks.

Strain with cheesecloth and discard lavender flowers and vanilla beans. Add the vegetable glycerin, vanilla extract and lavender essential oil to the reserved liquids and blend well. Put lid back onto jar and allow it to age for six weeks. Strain the perfume once again through a coffee filter then transfer it to a nice looking decorative spray bottle.

Shea Butter Deodorant

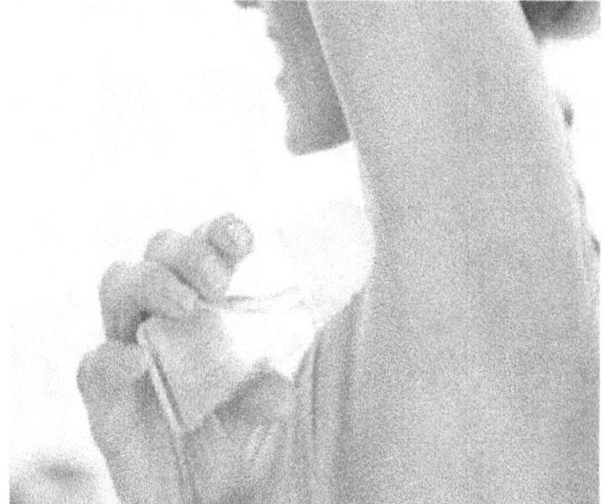

Ingredients:

- two tablespoons of Arrowroot powder

- three tablespoons of baking soda

- two tablespoons of Shea butter

- three tablespoons of coconut oil

- Essential oil of your choice

Directions:

In a double broiler over medium heat melt your Shea butter and coconut oil. Combine them in a mason jar placing into the broiler. Remove from heat and add in your arrowroot and baking soda.

Mix well. Add in your choice of essential oils. Pour into a glass container to store. You do not have to refrigerate. You may choose to put it into an old deodorant stick once it has cooled completely for easier use. You can speed up the hardening process by putting it into the fridge

Avocado shampoo

This recipe is made to make your hair look clean and fresh. It will also remove oil from the scalp. This shampoo is the best example that will not only nurture your hair, but it will also reduce oil production.

Ingredients:

1 cup organic castile soap

1 avocado (ripe)

Two teaspoons baking soda

¼ cup Luke warm water (distil water)

Recipe:

Take an avocado, peel it and put it in the blender. Run the blender and make a smooth puree. Add castile soap and baking soda into it and blend it again till a smooth mixture is formed. The mixture will be a thick paste. Start adding small amount of water bit by bit and blend it. Keep on adding small amount of water till you get the desired consistency. Take out all the material and store it in an airtight container. The shelf life of this mixture is 2 weeks.

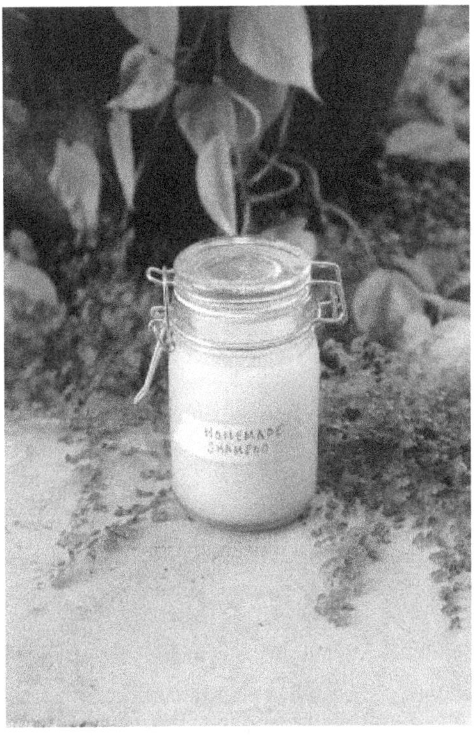

Heal Dry Cracked Feet

Make a balm for dry cracked feet by mixing a few drops (maximum 3) of lavender oil in coconut oil (2 tablespoons). Apply before going to bed.

Aromatherapy for Beautiful Skin: Reduce Age Spots

Apply frankincense oil on your age spots and sun spots on your skin thrice a day.

Natural Skin Toner

Make a 2% solution of frankincense, geranium, and lavender oils with water i.e. two drops of each oil in eight ounces of water. Keep this mix in a bottle. Apply on your skin before makeup every day.

Healing Salve

Ingredients:

- sixteen ounces of base oil such as almond oil, coconut oil or olive oil

- one and a half ounces of beeswax

- essential oils chosen by you for their particular healing properties

When you are making homemade herbal salves they usually include fat carrier oil and herbal oils. The essential oils you choose will be added after the process of heating the base oil, or infused oil with beeswax. After this has been removed from heat then the essential oils are added.

Supplies you will need to make your herbal salves are:

- herb infused oil with desired herbs of your choice

- beeswax

- jars or tins to store your salve in

- cheesecloth to drain out oil and separate herbs from oil

- essential oils that you choose to you in your salve

Choosing Herbs for Your Salve:

To begin the first thing that you must decide is what particular herbs you want to use to make your infused herbal oil. Take precaution when handling the ingredients. Do not overwhelm yourself when you are trying to decide what herbs you want to include in your infused oil. You would be best to start with 3-5 herbs. It is a very good idea to do the research and make sure that they are compatible with any medications that you are taking.

Making Your Herbal Infused Oil: Once you have chosen the herbs that you are going to use to make your herbal infused oil the next thing you must do in the process is to choose what kind of carrier oil you are going to use. I myself prefer to use coconut oil for my salves because it has great properties and is nice and firm. Sometimes I will mix it with a bit of olive oil as this is great for the skin.

When you have decided how much product you are making this will help you to decide on the size of containers you will need in order to store it in. I like to use small canning jars as they are perfect for when you have to put them into a double broiler to heat them. Fill your canning jars half-full of herbs. I will add more of my key herb than the rest of them.

Now add in your choice of carrier oil to heat-proof bowl along with the herbs. Heat over low heat in a double broiler with water half-way up the outside of the bowl that contains the oil and herbs. Heat oil for about three hours then allow to cool and stress oil through cheesecloth into another collection container. Discard the herbs. Add the oil back into the heat-proof bowl with beeswax and heat until the wax has melted. Add into your choice of storage containers that have secure lids.

<u>***Basic Body Spray***</u>

8 oz. of distilled water (distilled water is boiled and the steam is collected in a clean container; this removes most impurities)

1 Table Spoon of witch hazel (witch hazel takes the place of alcohol, it is gentler and has skin soothing properties)

20 -30 drops of essential oil

A spray pump bottle that will hold 8 oz. or more

Directions:

In the spray bottle, mix the distilled water with the witch hazel, and then add the essential oil/oils. Make sure the pump is on tight and shake the mixture well. Essential oil does not blend with water, it eventually separates, you will have to shake your spray before each use.

The following are recipes for body sprays, each recipe has different parts of essential oil added to the basic body spray:

Uplifting and Energizing: 5 drops of lavender oil and 15 drops of grapefruit oil.

Cozy and Romantic: 10 drops of cinnamon leaf oil and 15 drops of sweet orange oil.

Concentration and Focus: 5 drops of rosemary oil, 10 drops of peppermint oil, and 10 drops of patchouli oil.

Romantic Evening: 15 drops of rose oil and 10 drops of ylang-ylang.

Sweet Dreams: 15 drops of lavender oil and 10 drops of roman chamomile oil.

Winter Wonderland: 5 drops of vanilla oil (vanilla extract), 10 drops of cinnamon leaf oil, and 10 drops of sweet orange oil.

Banish the Blues: 10 drops of lavender oil and 10 drops of lemon oil.

Final Exam Focus Potion: 5 drops of lemon oil, 5 drops of black pepper oil, and 10 drops of peppermint oil.

Confident and Calm: 10 drops of rosemary oil, 5 drops of grapefruit oil, and 10 drops of geranium oil.

Peaceful Joy: 10 drops of frankincense oil and 10 drops of geranium oil.

Daydream Bliss: 10 drops of tea tree oil, 10 drops of lavender oil, and 5 drops of geranium oil.

Now that you have an idea of how much to use you should experiment with combinations of your own. You can begin by changing the amounts in these recipes to see what affect it has on the scent. Everyone is different, you may prefer more lavender and less tea tree in the Daydream Bliss recipe, so play around with the scents and amounts.

Solid Organic Perfume

Ingredients:

- two tablespoons of beeswax
- 35 drops of lavender essential oil
- two tablespoons of olive oil

Directions:

In a double broiler add in your wax stir until melted then remove from heat. Add in the oils and pour into final container.

To use this wonderful solid perfume just wipe it on the interior of your wrist this will leave a wonderful clean scent that will last all day!

Clay Shampoo:

This recipe will remove oil from the scalp. Clay has the property that it can absorb oil very well. It also contains minerals that are good for your scalp. Green tea contains antioxidants. It is also good for controlling dandruff and has an antibacterial effect. You need to store them in plastic air tight container. It is not recommended to store them in a metal container. Putting them in a metal container can produce a chemical reaction which can destroy the quality of the shampoo.

- Ingredients:

- 1 tablespoon clay

- 1 tablespoon liquid soap

- 2 teaspoon green tea

- 10 drops of tea tree oil

Recipe:

Take all the ingredients and mix them together until it is green and muddy in consistency. Now you can apply this shampoo over your scalp and keep it for 15 minutes. Then apply water and make lather and rinse it off with the help of water.

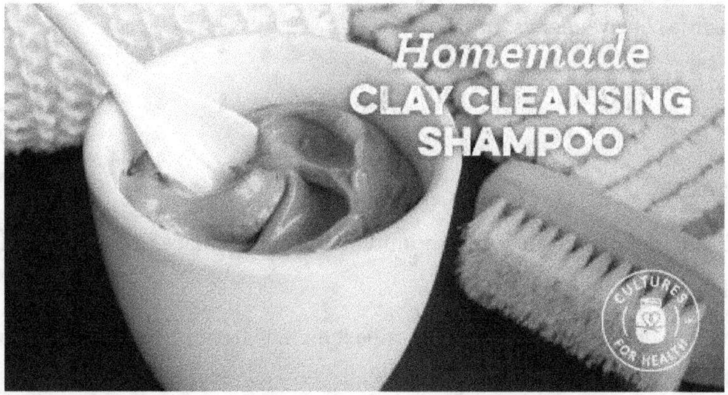

Vitamin E Deodorant

Ingredients:

- two tablespoons of cornstarch

- three tablespoons of Shea butter

- three tablespoons of baking soda

- two vitamin E caps

- two tablespoons of cocoa butter

- essential oil of your choice, about 15-20 drops

Directions:

Melt all of your ingredients except for the essential oil, and mix well. Remove from heat and add in the essential oil, mix well. Put into glass jar and allow to set in the refrigerator.

Facial Scrub

Mix five drops of lavender, grapefruit, and patchouli oils with one-fourth cup of cornmeal and one-fourth cup of yogurt. Apply this paste on your face. Let it dry. Rinse thoroughly with lukewarm water.

Reduce Stretch Marks:

Make a solution of a few drops (maximum five) of grapefruit, myrrh, and frankincense oils with coconut oil. Keep this cream in a container in the refrigerator. Apply it on the stretch marks as often as you desire.

Reduce Wrinkles

Mix a few drops (maximum three each) of frankincense, lavender, geranium, and sandalwood oils with any unscented lotion. Keep this in a container. Apply this cream on your washed face before going to bed. Avoid contact with eyes.

Orange & Wintergreen Creamy Body Salve

Ingredients:

- one cup of coconut butter

- half a cup of coconut oil

- half a cup of Jojoba oil

- twelve drops of orange essential oil

- twelve drops of wintergreen essential oil

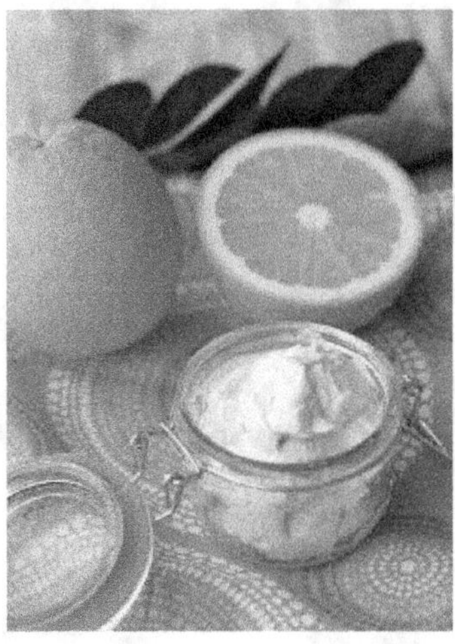

Directions:

Melt the coconut butter along with coconut oil and Jojoba oil, in a double broiler over medium heat. Once it is melted remove from heat and add in your essential oils and blend well.

Place mix into the fridge until it is almost hard, remove and whip with hand mixer until fluffy. Place in container for storage and put back into fridge for another ten minutes. Remove from fridge and secure on the lid. Store this salve for up to ten months. It will work great on sore aching muscles and dry skin.

Basic homemade jar deodorant for sensitive skin

1/3 cup of coconut oil – coconut oil is great for making deodorant, it solidifies and is wonderful for your skin, it moisturizes and its anti-oxidant properties help stop skin irritation.

2 table spoons of baking soda – baking soda corrects and helps maintain proper ph balance and absorbs odors.

1/3 of arrow root powder – this is used as a thickener to thicken the deodorant paste.

10-15 drops of essential oil – you can choose any essential oil you like or you can mix oils for a special blend.

Directions:

Mix the coconut oil, baking soda, and arrow root powder together in a mixing bowl. Continue to blend the ingredients until it has a deodorant type consistency.

Blend in the essential oil/oils

Put the deodorant into a glass container with a wide mouth. The wide mouth makes it easy to use your fingers to apply it. Glass is also easier to clean oil from than plastic so you can reuse the container when you need more deodorant.

Try using the essential oil blends you use for your body spray so you can reinforce the scent. Create a stress reducing deodorant for stressful busy days to keep you cool, calm, and collected.

Panthenol Shampoo:

This shampoo is devised to reduce the oil production from your scalp thus; it is very good for oily hair. The main ingredient of panthenol is very effective in reducing oil from the scalp. This shampoo is also very beneficial for the growth of new hair. The panthenol allows stiffness to hair shaft thus; decrease the amount of breaking of hair.

Ingredients:

- 2 cups Natural Nettle shampoo
- 2 tablespoon of panthenol shampoo
- 1 tablespoon of nettle extract
- 1 tablespoon of Vitamin B
- 2 tablespoon of castor oil

Recipe:

Take a bowl and mix all the ingredients together until a smooth mixture is formed. Put that in an air tight container.

Whenever, you go to take a bath. Wet your hair with the help of water. Take a small amount of this shampoo and massage it until lather is formed. Wash it with the help of water. You will see the effect with the first wash. New hair growth will bow visible within 3 to 4 months of use.

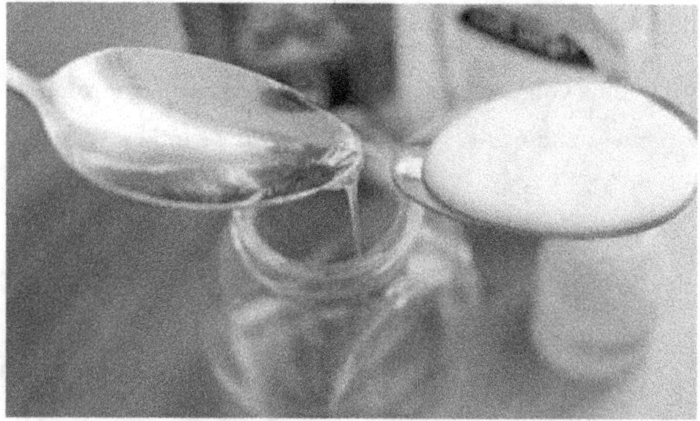

Simple Deodorant

Ingredients:

- one quarter cup of arrowroot powder

- five tablespoon of coconut oil

- one quarter cup of baking soda

Directions:

Mix arrowroot powder and baking soda then add in coconut oil mixing it into a paste. You can store in a small container or put into an empty deodorant stick for use.

Body Spray

Take a spray bottle. Pour a few drops (maximum ten each) of any essential oil of your preference in it. Add four ounces of water. Shake and spray on your skin. You can also mix two or more essential oils in it.

Sugar Scrub

Take any essential oil of your choice and mix a few drops of it in sugar and almond oil. Keep it in a container. Scrub your skin with it. You can also make sea salt scrub in the same way.

Homemade Deodorant

Take a spray bottle. Mix beeswax and coconut oil with any essential oil of your choice in it. According to the standards, you must mix clove and cedar wood oils for men and tea tree and lavender essential oils for women as a homemade deodorant.

Basic Calendula Salve

Ingredients:

- two and a half ounces of Calendula, dried

- six ounces of almond oil

- one quarter of a cup of beeswax

Directions:

Add all of your ingredients into a double broiler heating over simmer for three hours. Remove from heat and stress the oil using a cheesecloth. Discard the herbs and collect oil in container.

Add your collected herbal infused oil and put into heat-proof bowl along with beeswax and reheat in broiler over medium heat until the beeswax is melted. Allow to cool enough so then you can put into storage containers. Seal with secure lid. Store this salve in a cool dark place for up to a year.

Homemade stick deodorant for sensitive skin:

This deodorant is put into empty stick deodorant containers; these containers can be purchased online. This deodorant works just as good as the jar one but it is easier to use. You can add essential oils to this recipe too, just use 10-15 drops of your favorite scents.

- 1/3 cup of coconut oil

- 3 tablespoons of bees' wax, you can use pellets or grate it

- 2 tablespoons of shea butter

- 1/3 cup of arrowroot powder

- 2 tablespoons baking soda

- 10-15 drops of essential oil

Directions:

Heat the coconut oil, bees' wax and shea butter in a sauce pan. Stir continuously and keep the flame low. Heat until completely melted and blended.

Remove the saucepan from the heat and using a whisk, add the arrowroot powder and baking soda. Add the essential oil and mix it in well, do this quickly because the mixture begins to solidify quickly.

Fill 2 stick deodorant containers, Let the deodorant harden completely then put the lid on. Use this deodorant the same way you would use any store bought stick deodorant.

That's it, you are done. When you are deciding which oils to add to your deodorant, search through a list for essential oils that have deodorant properties. Adding essential oil with deodorant properties will make your homemade deodorant even better.

Raspberry & Lemon Body Mist

Ingredients:

- 25 raspberry essential oil drops
- 15 lemon essential oil drops
- half an ounce of witch hazel
- two tablespoons of vegetable glycerin
- distilled water

Directions:

Mix all ingredients in dark-glass spray bottle and shake before each and every use

Apple cider vinegar shampoo:

This shampoo with apple cider as the main ingredient is another addition to the list of shampoo for dry hair. Apple cider can clean all the dirt and wax from your hairs. Lemon has vitamin C which has antioxidant properties. The egg has a protein that will be beneficial for the life of your hair. This shampoo will leave your hair smooth, aft and nurtured.

Ingredients:

1 teaspoon apple cider vinegar

1 cup liquid soap

1 egg

2 tablespoon fresh lemon juice

1 tablespoon olive oil

Recipe:

Take a blender and start adding all the ingredients into it. Blend all the material until a smooth mixture is formed. Your shampoo is ready to be used. Take out all the mixture and put it in a glass bottle. This shampoo has a life of around 2 weeks.

When you go to take a bath, take a small amount of this shampoo and apply to your wet hair. Apply the shampoo and massage your hair for 3 to 5 minutes and produce a lot of lather. Rinse your hair with the help of water. You will feel your hair be healthier and smooth. With the use of 1 month, you will see a decrease in oil content of your hair.

DIY Natural Solid Deodorant

Ingredients:

- one tablespoon of beeswax

- two tablespoons of coconut oil

- one tablespoon of Shea butter

- three drops of Citronella essential oil

- three drops of lemongrass essential oil

- one tablespoon of baking soda

- one and a half tablespoons of Bentonite clay

- two tablespoons of arrowroot powder

- three drops of Tea tree essential oil

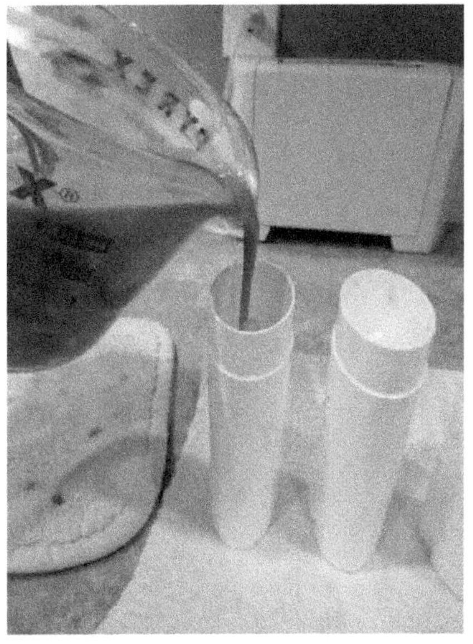

Directions:

In a double broiler add in your bees wax, coconut oil and Shea butter over medium heat stir until the wax and oils have melted. Remove mix from heat and add in your essential oils, arrowroot powder, Bentonite clay and mix well.

Pour this liquid into some silicone muffin molds or an empty deodorant container and allow to cool down and solidify for about three hours. The bees wax is going to help keep it solid so you can use it like a traditional deodorant.

Acne Face Wash

Make a paste of tea tree essential oil with raw honey. Keep this cream in the refrigerator. Rub it on your face every time you wash it. Rinse with warm water.

Natural Perfume

Simple rub two to three drops of jasmine essential oil on your wrist. You can also use lavender and vanilla essential oils in the same manner if you are a woman. For men, clove and cypress oils are the best options.

Reduce Cellulite

Make a paste by mixing a few drops of grapefruit essential oil and coconut oil. Keep it in a container. Massage it on the affected area often.

Lavender & Coconut Muscle Salve

Ingredients:

- half a cup of coconut oil

- three tablespoons of Shea butter

- one quarter of a cup of beeswax

- half a teaspoon of vitamin E oil

- 20 drops of lavender essential oil

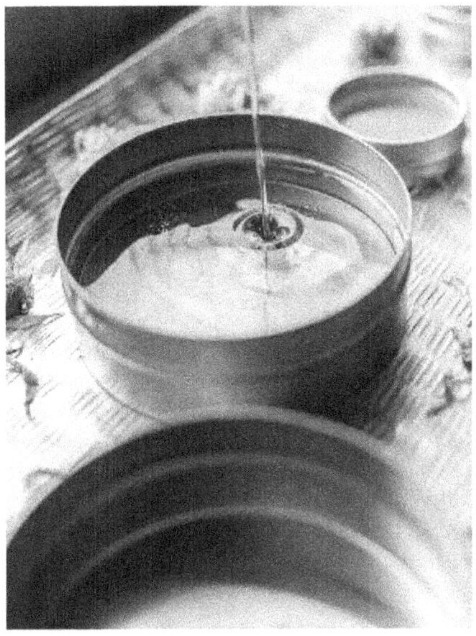

Directions:

In a double broiler over medium heat add in coconut oil, Shea butter and beeswax. Stir until it is melted then remove from heat. Add in the vitamin E oil and essential oil and mix well. Add to chosen storage containers and secure lid. You can store this salve up to six months.

Shea Butter Deodorant

- 3 tablespoons of coconut oil

- 3 tablespoons of baking soda

- 2 tablespoons of shea butter

- 2 tablespoons of arrowroot powder

- 10-15 drops of essential oil

Directions:

Place a glass container/mason jar/mixing bowl in a pot of hot water. Put the shea butter and coconut oil in the glass container and melt over a low flame and mix it together until completely blended.

Remove the mixture from the heat and add the baking soda and arrowroot. Mix until completely blended then add the essential oils and mix again.

Pour the mixture into a glass container with a lid, small mason jars work great for this. Wait until the mixture solidifies before you use it. You can store it in the fridge but it is not necessary, it will stay solid if stored at room temperature.

This deodorant is applied with your fingers, it is creamy and the shea butter is great for your skin.

Coconut shampoo

This shampoo is made up of coconut and essential oils. With the aid of this oil, the dry scalp can be treated, and dryness of hair will be taken off. The shelf life of this shampoo is around 1 week.

Ingredients:

- 1 cup coconut milk
- 1 cup aloe Vera gel
- 1 cup Essential oils (Vitamin E oil, jojoba oil, or sweet almond oil)

Recipe:

Take a bowl and add all the ingredients into it. Mix them until it is smooth with the help of a whisk. Pour this mixture into ice cube tray and put them in the freezer. You need to use this shampoo twice a week. Whenever you wish to take a bath, take one cube which will be sufficient for one wash.

Take that cube and apply it on the scalp and then towards the end of the hair. Wait for 30 seconds. This cube will not produce any lather. Apply it for a period of 15 minutes then rinse it off with water.

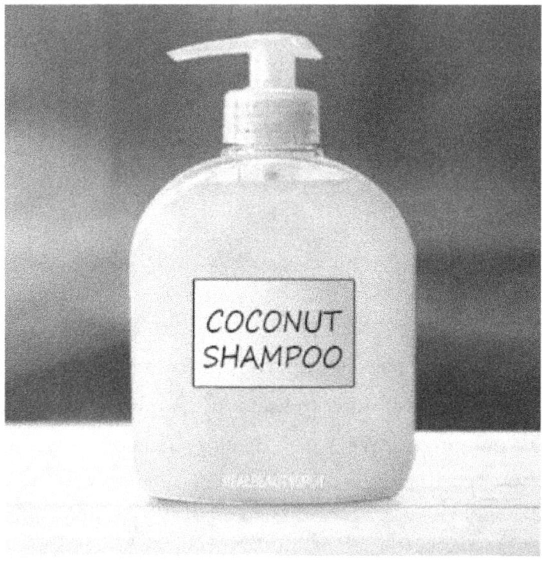

Natural Coconut Deodorant

Ingredients:

- one eighth of a cup of arrowroot powder
- one eighth of a cup of cornstarch
- one quarter of a cup of coconut oil
- one tablespoon of baking soda
- essential oils of your choice, about ten drops

Directions:

In a mixing bowl add cornstarch, coconut oil, baking soda, arrowroot powder and mix well. Add in your essential oils and mix.

Pour mix into an empty deodorant container or into a small mason jar and place in the fridge for twenty minutes. Remove from fridge as use as needed.

Oily Hair

Make a solution of a few drops (maximum ten) each of rosemary, lime, and ylang-ylang oils with any unscented oil (two ounces) and apply on your scalp thrice a week. Rinse out as usual.

Deep Hair Conditioner

Take lavender oil and sandalwood oil in equal quantity (maximum five drops each) and mix with 15 drops of rosewood oil. Mix this solution in any unscented oil. Put this cream in a plastic bag and place that bag in warm water to heat it up. Apply warm cream in your hair. Leave in for at least 20 minutes. Wash with regular shampoo.

Cure Dandruff

Make a solution of a few drops (maximum five each) of lavender and rosemary oils with unscented oil (maximum three tablespoons). Apply this solution on your scalp. Leave in for at least ten minutes. Rinse using shampoo as usual.

Spearmint Pain Reliever Salve

Ingredients:

- half a cup of coconut oil

- two ounces of beeswax

- 15 drops of cinnamon essential oil

- 20 drops of camphor essential oil

- 20 drops of spearmint essential oil

- eight drops of clove essential oil

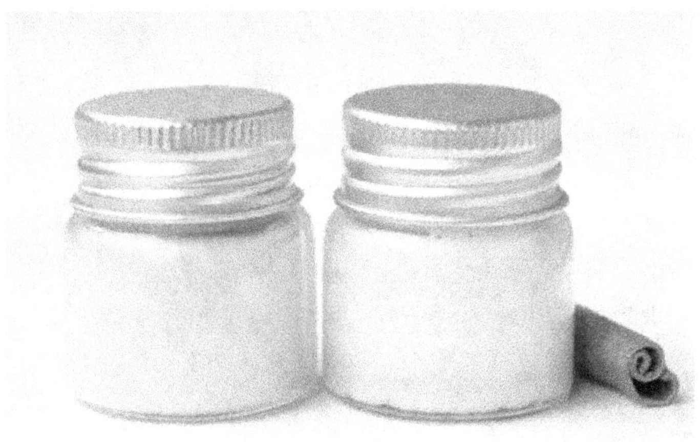

Add to your double broiler the coconut oil, and beeswax over medium heat, stir until mix is melted. Remove from the heat and add in your essential oils and blend mix well. Add to tins or jars and seal lid. Allow to cool before you use it. This is a great salve that will help relieve pain in sore muscles and even headaches.

Coconut Oil Deodorant:

This deodorant uses coconut oil instead of shea butter and coconut oil. It works just as well as the other deodorants. You can adjust the powder ingredients to get the consistency you want for your deodorant. It is creamy when finished and you apply it with your fingertips.

- 6 tablespoons of coconut oil

- 4 tablespoons of baking soda

- 4 teaspoons of arrowroot or cornstarch

- 10-15 drops of essential oil

Directions:

Mix the baking soda and arrowroot/cornstarch in a bowl.

Add the coconut oil to the baking soda and arrowroot mixture and blend it together using the back side of a spoon or a fork. Make sure it is completely blended together then add the essential oil and blend again.

Put the finished mixture into a small glass container with a lid. A small mason jar work for this. Let the deodorant sit until it is firm, apply with fingertips.

Cucumber shampoo

This shampoo is the answer to your dry hair and scalp. It has integrated cleansing property of lemon and nurturing property of cucumber that will not only give life to you hair but also treat your dry hair. All you need to do is make this shampoo and wash you hair every time with it.

Ingredients:

- 1 cucumber
- 2 tablespoon lemon juice
- 1 cup liquid soap

Recipe:

Peel the cucumber and blend it in a blender so that a smooth paste is formed. Now add lemon juice and liquid soap to the blender. Blend all the ingredients till a smooth paste is formed. Store this shampoo in an air tight container and refrigerate it. This shampoo will last for 2 weeks.

When you go to take a bath, take a small amount of this shampoo and wet your hair. Apply the shampoo and massage your hair for 3 to 5 minutes. A lot of lather will be formed. Rinse your hair with the help of water. You will feel your hair be healthier and smooth. With the use of 1 month, you will see a decrease in oil content of your hair.

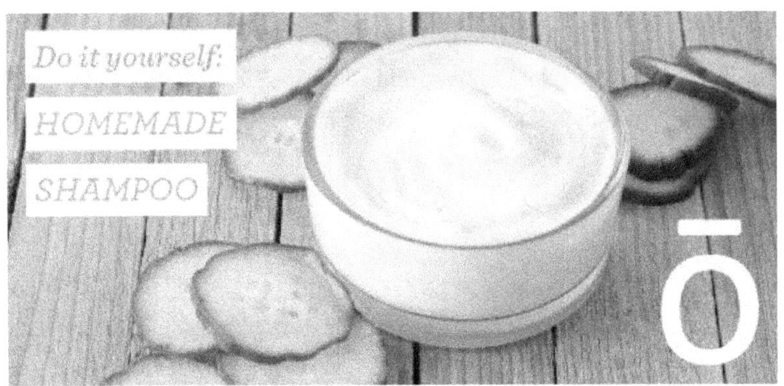

Detoxifying Natural Deodorant

Ingredients:

- two tablespoons of Bentonite clay

- four tablespoons of arrowroot powder

- four tablespoons of baking soda

- six tablespoons of coconut oil

- 20 drops of Tea tree essential oil

Directions:

Add all of your ingredients into a mixing bowl and blend well. Heat the coconut oil first so that it will mix easily with other ingredients. Knead the mixture with your hands to make it into a smooth paste.

Add to empty deodorant stick or glass jar. Allow it to cool. Scoop out with finger when you want to apply the paste. Rub paste under arms it will melt quickly into your skin.

Thicken Hair

Take the bottle of your regular shampoo and add a few drops of rosemary essential oil in it. Shampoo your hair with it every time you wash your hair.

Itchy Scalp

Take the bottle of your regular shampoo and add a few drops of basil, cedarwood, and lavender essential oils in it. Keep it with you. Shampoo your hair with it every time you wash your hair.

Homemade Shampoo

Make a shampoo type paste by mixing coconut milk, aloe vera gel, rosemary oil, and lavender oil. Keep it in a bottle. Use this shampoo every time you wash your hair. It will last for three to four weeks.

Arnica Pain Relieving Salve

Ingredients:

- one cup of coconut oil

- one ounce of Arnica, dried

- one quarter of a teaspoon of vitamin E

- 20 drops of Marjoram essential oil

- one quarter of a cup of beeswax

Directions:

In a double broiler add your coconut oil, along with the Arnica and simmer for two hours. Remove from heat and stress the oil using a cheesecloth. Collect oil in container and discard the herbs.

Add oil along with beeswax back into broiler over medium heat, stir until melted. Remove from heat and add in your essential oil and vitamin E and mix well. Add mix to containers and seal lid. Keep in a dark cool place, this salve will last for up to a year. It works well for aching muscles and bones.

Vitamin E and Shea Butter Deodorant:

Vitamin E and shea butter are fabulous skin conditioners and moisturizers. This deodorant uses vitamin E and shea butter in a mix that keeps odors away and cares for the sensitive skin under your arms. This recipe makes 4oz of deodorant.

- 30g of coconut oil

- 20g of shea butter

- 10g of almond oil

- 10g of bees' wax

- 15g of arrowroot powder

- 15g of food grade diatomaceous earth

- 5 drops of vitamin E

- 10-15 drops of essential oil

Directions:

Place a glass container in a pot of hot water over a low flame, add the coconut oil, shea butter, bees' wax, almond oil, vitamin E oil, and the essential oil and mix as it melts, the bees' wax will take longer to melt and blend in.

Once the oils and wax are blended well, remove from heat and let cool a few minutes. Add the dry ingredients and use a whisk to blend everything together.

Pour the mixture into a small glass container with a lid, a small masons jar will do fine. Allow the mixture to set and solidify before you use it. Use your fingertips to apply the deodorant.

All of these deodorants work great. If you are sensitive to any of them try removing the baking soda. For many, baking soda is the reason for the sensitivity. If you are still sensitive discontinue use and see if the problem corrects itself.

There are many essential oils with deodorant properties, try adding one of these along with the fragrance you like. You can break down the 10-15 drops of essential oil and us several to create a blended fragrance that is uniquely yours. You can even use the same essential oils in your deodorant that you use in your body spray for a longer lasting scent.

Tea tree oil shampoo

This shampoo is a mixture of honey, apple cider vinegar, tea tree oil and green tea. Tea tree oil is beneficial for oil control as it can unblock sebum that is blocking your hair follicles. It also has antibacterial and anti fungal properties. Honey makes hair smooth and soft. It also has antibacterial properties. Apple cider vinegar has the anti bacterial property that can kill oil producing bacteria.

Ingredients:

- 2 tablespoon castile soap
- 1 tablespoon honey
- 2 tablespoon apple cider vinegar
- 10 drops tea tree oil
- 3 tablespoon green tea
- Half cup water (preferably distil water)

Recipe:

Take a bowl and mix all the ingredients except water and tea tree oil. Now add tea tree oil. Mix well so that a smooth mixture is formed. Make sure there are no lumps in it. At this moment, the mixture will be quite thick. To reduce its thickness adds a small amount of water till it gets off the consistency of shampoo. Take a container and store i in that container preferably glass container.

When you go to take a bath, Rinse your hair with water so that they are wet. Take small amount f this shampoo and apply on your scalp. Rub them till a lot of lather is formed. Rub your hair for five minutes. Now wash your hair with water.

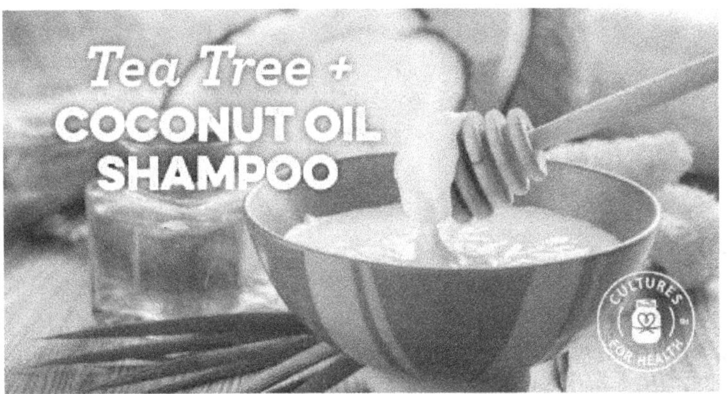

Rubbing Alcohol

Ingredients:

- Rubbing alcohol

- cotton balls

- optional 20 drops of your choice of essential oil

Directions:

You can kill the odor causing bacteria by using this inexpensive way of helping to fight this problem. Just fill a spray bottle with rubbing alcohol then spritz your underarms, or you can choose to dab it on with a cotton ball.

You can also add some of your favorite essential oil to make it smell more pleasing.

Basic Comfrey Salve

Ingredients:

- two and a half ounces of comfrey leaves, dried

- one cup of almond oil

- one quarter of a cup of beeswax

- twelve drops of Camphor essential oil

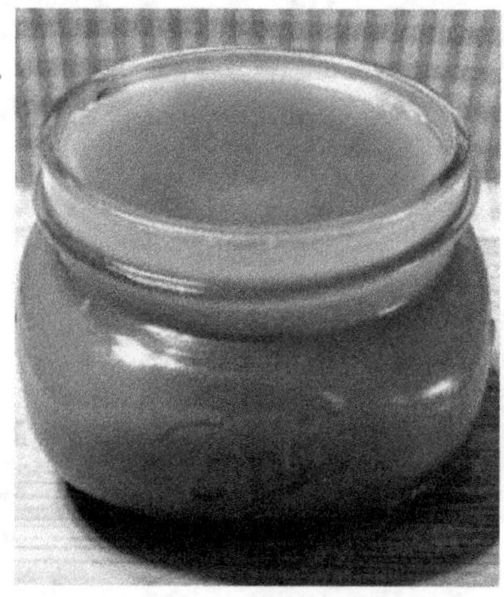

Directions:

Place the comfrey leaves and almond oil into double broiler over simmer for an hour. Remove from heat and stress the oil through cheesecloth. Collect oil and discard the herbs. Add oil back into the double broiler with beeswax over medium heat, stir until melted.

Remove from heat add in the essential oil and mix well. Add mix to containers and seal with secure lid. This is a great salve to help with skin wounds, or skin problems. First clean wound with hydrogen peroxide then apply the salve.

African black soap shampoo:

This soap contains natural ingredient which includes palm leaves, plantain skin an ash, cocoa pod ash, shea butter and palm kernel oil. Honey or glycerin can lock moisture in your hair. All you need to do is go to the kitchen and have these items and make your shampoo out of natural products.

Ingredients:

- 4 tablespoon of African black soap
- 2 teaspoon glycerin
- 3 teaspoon essential oil (preferably grape seed oil)

Recipe:

Take 4 tablespoons of African black soap. Crumble it into small pieces. Add this into the blender. Now add other ingredients to the blender. Blend it till a smooth mixture is formed. Your African soap shampoo is ready to be used.

Use it while taking a bath. This shampoo can be saved for a couple of weeks.

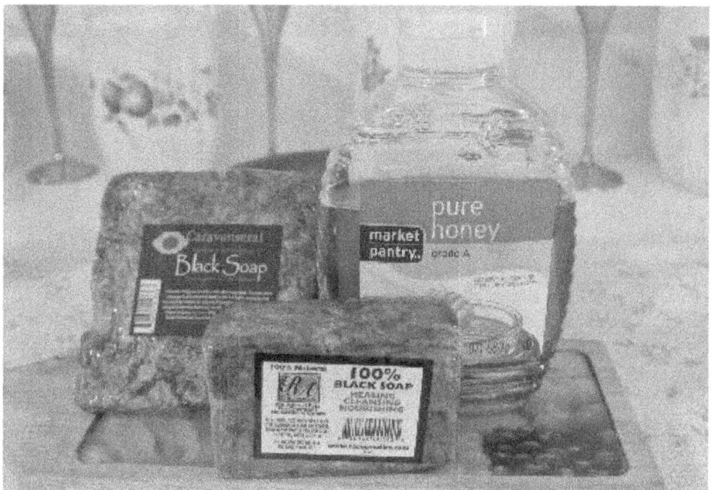

Lemon Juice Deodorant

Ingredients:

- lemon juice

Directions:

Lemon juice is a great natural deodorizer that many people enjoy making use of. In the lemon juice is citric acid that helps to kill the odor-causing bacteria under your arms. Use a slice of lemon on your armpits in the morning. You may also collect the juice in a spray bottle and spritz the juice on to your underarms. Keep in mind not to use the lemon juice on areas that have recently been shaved.

All-Natural Homemade Deodorant

Ingredients:

- one eighth of a cup of arrowroot powder

- one eighth of a cup of cocoa butter

- half a tablespoon of baking soda

- six drops of vitamin E oil

- one eighth of cup of Shea Butter

- 25 drops of your choice of essential oil

Directions:

Combine your cocoa butter and Shea butter, mix well. Use a double broiler to heat oil over medium heat until they have become melted, blend well. Remove them from heat add in your baking soda, arrowroot powder, vitamin E and essential oil and mix well. Pour mix into two ounce tins, place lid gently on the top do not lock lid at this point. This is just to prevent dust from getting into the mixture while it is in the cooling down process. Leave it to cool down overnight.

Cracked Foot Heel Salve

Ingredients:

- one quarter of a cup of coconut oil

- one quarter of a cup of Shea butter

- one quarter of a cup of Magnesium flakes with two tablespoons of boiling water

- twelve drops of oregano essential oil

- fifteen drops of peppermint essential oil

Directions:

In a small bowl add two tablespoons of boiling water and add in the Magnesium flakes and mix. Allow to cool. In a double broiler add in the Shea butter, beeswax, and coconut oil, stir until melted over medium heat. Remove from heat and add into a bowl and blend well. Add in the Magnesium paste.

After it as been well-blended put into the fridge for twenty minutes. Remove from fridge and re-blend mix. Store mix for up to eight weeks in the fridge. Use this salve on dry or cracked feet at night. For the best results you should first exfoliate the skin from your feet before you apply the salve. Repeat this process until your feet are cleared up.

Cognac shampoo

This shampoo has cognac and egg main ingredient. Both of these ingredients have a good amount of protein. This adds life to your hair. It also allows new hair to grow. The egg helps you to lock the natural oil of the hair.

- 1 cup baby shampoo
- Half cup of cognac
- 1 tablespoon of honey
- 1 egg

Recipe:

Take all the ingredients and add them in a blender. Blend them all till a smooth mixture comes out. Now your cognac shampoo is ready to be used. Keep this in air tight container for use.

Whenever you want to take a bath, Rinse your hair with water so that they are wet. Take small amount f this shampoo and apply on your scalp. Rub them till a lot of lather is formed. Rub your hair for five minutes. Now wash your hair with water.

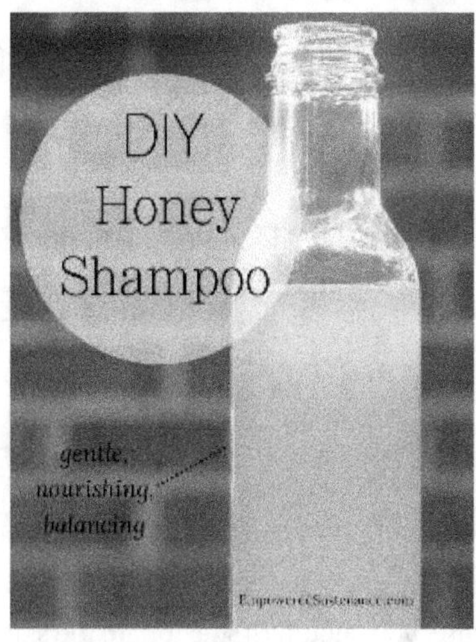

Summertime Deodorant

Ingredients:

- one quarter of cup of baking soda
- one quarter of a cup of cornstarch
- four tablespoons of coconut oil
- one and a half tablespoons of bees wax, grated
- six Tea tree essential oil drops
- six drops of lavender essential oil

Directions:

Melt your oils in a double broiler over medium heat and stir until melted. Remove from heat then add in the rest of your ingredients. Mix well. Add this paste into an empty deodorant container.

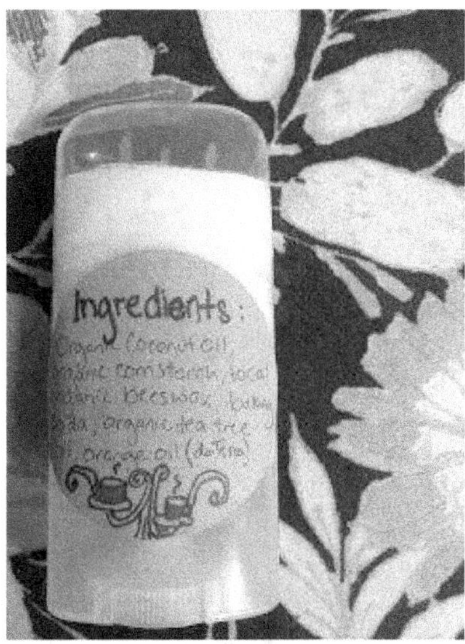

Calendula & Comfrey Salve

Ingredients:

- half an ounce of Calendula, dried
- half an ounce of Comfrey, dried
- one cup of cold pressed olive oil
- half an ounce of beeswax
- five vitamin E capsules

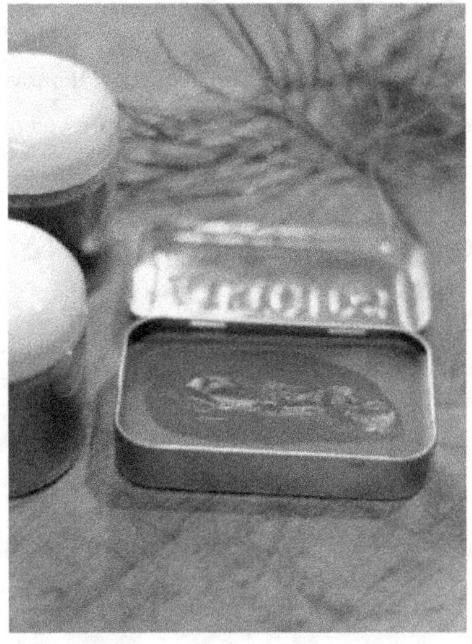

Directions:

In your double broiler add in oil and herbs cook on low for 30 minutes, stirring occasionally. Allow the mix to cool then stress it through cheesecloth collect oil and discard the herbs. Add collected oil back into the double broiler with beeswax and over medium heat stir until melted. Remove from heat and add in vitamin E capsules. Add to jars and seal with secure lid.

Castile Shampoo:

This shampoo is all set to go for normal hair. Castile is the soap that is made up f olive oil that is all natural. You can use this shampoo two times a week that will save and add life to your hair.

Ingredients:

- Half cup Castile flakes
- 1-liter water
- ¼ cup olive oil

Recipe:

All you need is to take a pan. Put 1-liter water into it. Turn it to boil. Take Castile flakes in a bowl and now pour this water over the flakes. Now add olive oil into it. Add all the ingredients and mix them well to make a smooth mixture. Now your Castile shampoo is all ready to be used. Keep it and store in a glass bottle. This shampoo will work for a couple of weeks.

Whenever you want to take a bath, Rinse your hair with water so that they are wet. Take small amount f this shampoo and apply on your scalp. Rub them till a lot of lather is formed. Rub your hair for five minutes. Now wash your hair with water.

Deodorant Bar

Ingredients:

- half a cup of Shea butter

- half a cup of coconut butter

- half a cup of bees wax

- three tablespoons of baking soda

- one and a half teaspoons of vitamin E oil

- three capsules of high quality probiotics

- half a cup of arrowroot powder

- 25 drops of essential oil of your choice

Directions:

In a double broiler add in the Shea butter, coconut oil, and beeswax, over medium heat stir until melted. Remove from heat and add in your arrowroot powder, vitamin E, probiotics, baking soda, and essential oil, mix well. Just make sure before adding these ingredients that the oil is not too hot.

You do not want to kill your probiotics. Gently stir the mix until well blended. Pour int
muffin tins or another mold that can hold liquid. If you want to put it into an empty
deodorant stick then let it harden in bowl until it turns to be the consistency of peanut
butter. Add into empty deodorant stick, scooping and packing it down. Allow cover of
stick to stay off overnight to allow it to harden.

Polk Root & Blood Root Salve to Help in Treating Skin Cancer

Ingredients:

- one tablespoon of Polk root

- one tablespoon of Blood-Root

- one tablespoon of activated charcoal powder

- one tablespoon of Pascalite clay

- one tablespoon of almond oil

- one tablespoon of zinc chloride, crystal or liquid

- one teaspoon of wood tar

Directions:

Add two tablespoons of warm water if you are using the crystal form of zinc chloride an
mix until dissolved then set aside. Mix blood-root and Polk-root with almond oil and
charcoal powder. Add in the zinc and mix well. Heat mix in a double broiler for 30
minutes on low heat. Add in the Pascalite clay and wood tar, mix well into a paste.

If it seems too thick just add in a couple of more drops of almond oil. Apply this salve to
the area of skin that has cancer lesions and cover with a gauze for 12 hours. After the
treatment wash the area with soap and water then clean with hydrogen peroxide. Apply
this treatment every 2-3 days. The cancer lesions may disappear after one to five
months. You may experience stinging or burning this is normal.

Rosemary shampoo:

This rosemary shampoo is all set for normal hair. It will not only clean your hair, but it will also give your hair a lustrous shine. It will also provide freshness and life to your hair.

Ingredients:

- ¼ cup castile soap
- 2 tablespoon rosemary
- ¼ cup distils water
- 2 tablespoon almond oil
- ½ teaspoon lemon essential oil
-

Recipe:

Take a pan and add distil water into it. Bring water to boil. Take rosemary in a bowl and now add this water to the rosemary. Keep it submerged till the water gets cool to Luke warm temperature. Strain this water and the filtrate will be your base in which you will add the other entire ingredient. Now add castile soap, almonds oil and lemon essential oil to Luke warm water. Mix all the ingredients until a smooth mixture is formed. Your rosemary shampoo is ready to be used. Keep it in a glass jar to increase its life.

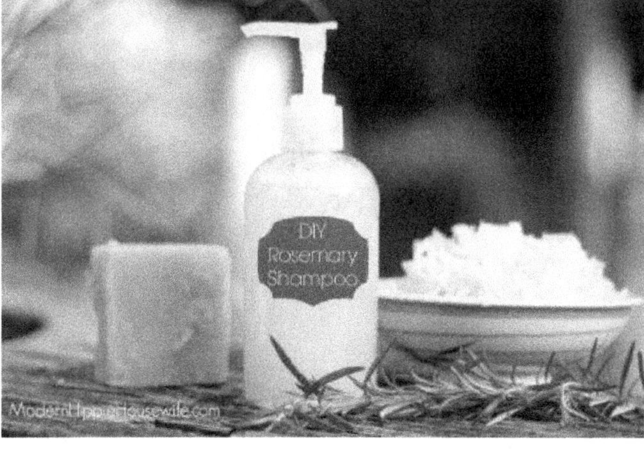

Homemade Deodorant

Ingredients:

- half a cup of baking soda

- half a cup of coconut oil

- 40 drops of your choice of essential oil

- empty deodorant container

Directions:

Put your oil into a bowl and mix baking soda into it. Add in the essential oil and blend well. Fill up the empty deodorant container with mix and leave out overnight with cap off to allow mix to harden.

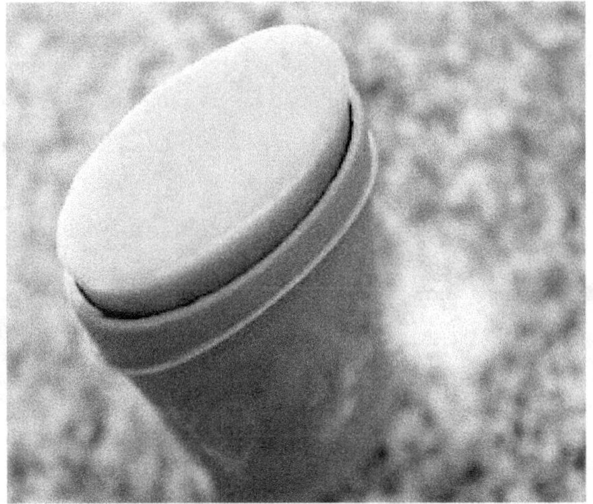

Blood-Root Black Salve for Skin Cancer

Ingredients:

- half a cup of blood-root, powdered

- half a cup of white flour

- half a cup of zinc chloride, crystals or liquid

- two cups of hot water

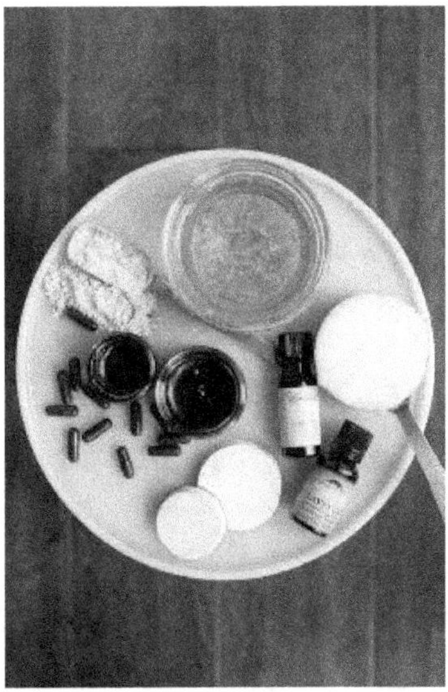

Directions:

Add all of your ingredients and mix except for water. Add to double broiler mix and water and mix well. This is a treatment used for skin cancer lesions. This is a good treatment for the skin cancer lesions that are at the top of the skin or exposed.

Once the mix has cooled then apply to area on skin where the cancer is. Do not try to pull off lesions they will fall out in 10 days time. You can add Vaseline around the outer rim of where you applied the salve so the mix does not irritate your surrounding skin.

Egg shampoo:

This shampoo is very easy to make. You do not need to go to buy anything from the market. All the ingredients are present in your kitchen. All you need to grab those and convert them into your shampoo. It is a moisturizing shampoo that will add life to your hair. Egg contains protein that is good for the health of the hair and it also locks the moisture in the hair.

Ingredients:

- 1 cup Castile liquid soap
- 2 eggs
- 3 teaspoon baking soda
- 2 teaspoon olive oil
- 2 teaspoon lemon juice
-

Recipe:

Beat the eggs and then add 1 cup of Castile liquid soap and add all the other ingredients into it. Blend all the material so that a smooth mixture is formed. Your egg shampoo is ready to be used.

Homemade Deodorant for Sensitive Skin

Ingredients:

- one quarter of a cup of Diatomaceous Earth (Food Grade)
- three quarters of a cup of arrowroot powder
- ten tablespoons of melted coconut oil

Directions:

Combine the arrowroot powder with the diatomaceous earth. Mix and keep adding in the melted oil a little at a time. Store in a small glass jar with secure lid use when needed by applying a small amount to your underarms.

Healing Echinacea Root Salve

Ingredients:

- one cup of almond oil

- one teaspoon of plantain leaf

- one teaspoon of echinacea root

- one quarter of a cup of beeswax

- one teaspoon of Calendula flowers

- one teaspoon of comfrey leaf

- one teaspoon of rosemary leaf

- one tablespoon of grapefruit seed extract

- one teaspoon of yarrow flowers

- twelve drops of peppermint essential oil

Directions:

In a double broiler add in almond oil and herbs in a heat-proof bowl, water should be in broiler halfway up the outside of the bowl. Heat your oil and herbs over low heat for three hours. Allow to cool so that you are able to stress the oil with cheesecloth, collect oil in a container then discard the herbs.

 Add the oil back into heat-proof bowl along with beeswax, reheat over medium heat until the beeswax is melted. Remove from heat and add in your essential oils and mix well. Pour into small containers this salve works well on dry and chapped lips.

Honey body wash:

With ingredients like honey, essential oils, and vitamin E oil, it is the best products that a good Homemade Body Wash for Dry Skin can have. Honey helps to retain moisture and elasticity of the skin. It can be used to treat itchy and damaged skin as well. Oil maintains the moisture of the body as well. Vitamin E is not only good for moisture of the skin but also repair damaged skin. There is no use of water in the recipe which gives it an advantage of the shelf life of up to a year.

Ingredients:

- 1 cup Castile liquid soap
- 3 tablespoon honey
- 2 teaspoon oil (jojoba, sweet almond, grape seed, sesame, or olive)
- 1 teaspoon vitamin E oil
- 2 teaspoon of essential oil (Chamomile, Geranium, Grapefruit, Lavender, Rosemary or Tea tree)

Recipe:

Take a blender and all the ingredients together. Blend them till a smooth mixture is formed. Store it in a beautiful glass jar for use.

When you go to take a bath, take a small amount of this on the wash cloth and use it.

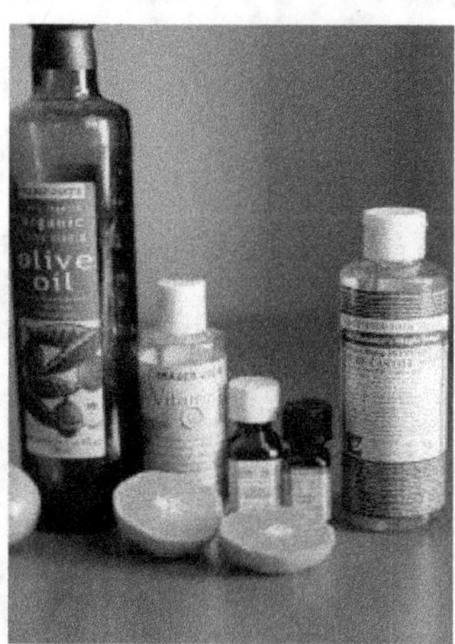

Sensitive Skin Deodorant

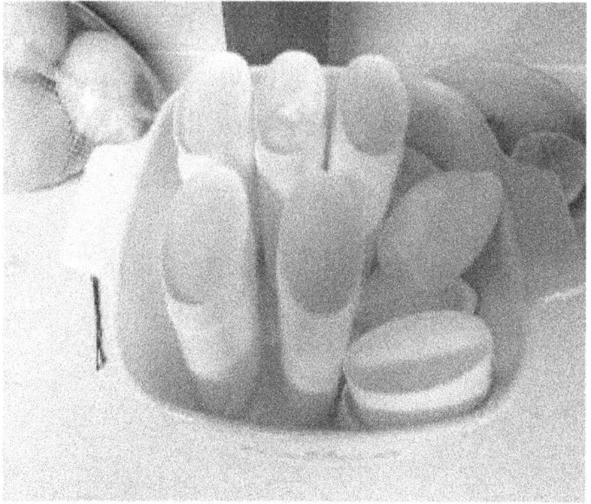

Ingredients:

- seven tablespoons of melted coconut oil

- one quarter of a cup of baking soda

- three quarters of a cup of cornstarch

Directions:

Combine your cornstarch with baking soda. Slowly add in the coconut oil a bit at a time blending it in as you go. Use a fork to help mash it down as you progress. Transfer mix to glass jar and seal with secure fitting lid. Apply a little using your fingertips as needed.

Pregnancy Stretch-Mark Salve

Ingredients:

- one quarter of a cup of almond oil

- one quarter of a cup of Shea butter

- five tablespoons of Apricot Kernel oil

- one tablespoon of Calendula flowers

- one quarter of a teaspoon of ginger-root, dried

Directions:

Add almond oil along with dry ginger-root, and Calendula flowers to double broiler in a heat-proof bowl. Simmer and mix for about three hours then remove from heat. Stress the oil in cheesecloth, collect oil in another container, discard the herbs.

Add the oil back into the heat-proof bowl add in the Shea butter and heat until the Shea butter is melted and mix well. Add mix to glass jar, this can be used during pregnancy and after.

Glycerin body wash:

This body wash with the addition of glycerin is an asset for dry skin. Castile soap is all natural and has no side effects at all. This body wash can be used without any problem. The best thing that you can have with this body wash is that 3 liters of body wash in just $4.5.

Ingredients:

- Castile soap
- 2 tablespoon glycerin
- 12 cups water

Recipe:

Take castile soap and grate it in small pieces with the help of grater. Take a pan and add 12 cups of water. Bring water to boil. Add this water to grated castile soap. Mix it till the soap melts and a mixture are formed. Add glycerin to it. Allow it to cool and set for almost 24 hours. Your body wash is ready to be used.

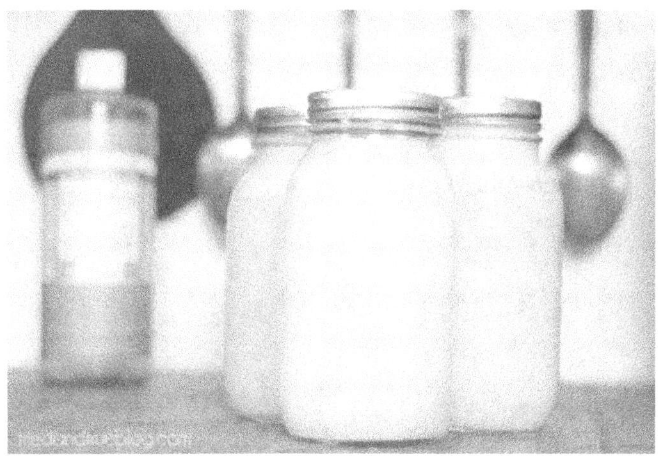

Coconut & Lavender Homemade Deodorant

Ingredients:

- seven tablespoons of coconut oil

- one quarter of a cup of arrowroot powder

- one quarter of a cup of baking soda

- 40 drops of lavender essential oil

Directions:

In a mixing bowl add baking soda, arrowroot powder, mix well, add in coconut oil and lavender essential oil slowly mashing with a fork. You can store the mix in an old deodorant container or in a small glass jar.

Orange Citrus Homemade Deodorant

Ingredients:

- one and a half teaspoons of bees wax, grated

- four tablespoons of coconut oil

- three tablespoons of Shea butter

- three tablespoons of arrowroot powder

- 35 drops of orange essential oil

Directions:

In a double broiler add in your bees wax, coconut oil and Shea butter, blend until melted. Remove from heat allow to cool down then add in orange essential oil, arrowroot powder and baking soda, blend well. Put mix in empty deodorant container or in small glass jar with secure lid. You can leave over night to allow to harden or you can speed this process up and put it in the fridge for 20 minutes.

Grapefruit Homemade Deodorant

Ingredients:

- four tablespoons of Shea butter

- two tablespoons of coconut oil

- one tablespoon of beeswax, grated

- four tablespoons of baking soda

- three tablespoons of arrowroot powder

- 40 drops of grapefruit essential oil

Directions:

In a double broiler add in your Shea butter, coconut oil, and beeswax stir until melted. Remove from heat allowing to cool then add in your baking soda, essential oils, and arrowroot powder mix well.

Add to empty deodorant container for easy use. You can speed up the hardening process by sticking it into the fridge for half an hour. Do not use on areas that have just been shaved.

Black-Drawing Salve

Ingredients:

- four tablespoons of comfrey
- three teaspoons of Shea butter
- three tablespoons of coconut oil
- one tablespoon of honey
- three tablespoons of Kaolin clay
- three tablespoons of Calendula, dried
- two tablespoons of charcoal powder, activated
- twenty drops of lavender essential oil
- two capsules of vitamin E

Directions:

Mix Calendula, comfrey and oil. Add to a jar and leave for five days. Each day shake the jar a few times a day. Then strain through a cheesecloth, discarding the herbs, and adding the infused oil to double broiler.

Add in also beeswax, Shea butter and vitamin E over medium heat until it is melted and mix well. Remove from heat and add in essential oil, charcoal powder, and kaolin clay and mix well. Store in glass jars that have secure lids. This salve works great on cuts and splinters.

Shea butter body wash:

This body wash includes shea butter which has ample amount of moisturizing oils. It is very good for itchy and tight skin.

Ingredients:

- Half cup cocoa butter
- 2 tablespoon shea butter
- 2 tablespoon coconut oil
- 2 tablespoon almond oil
- 1 tablespoon lemon juice
- Half cup castile soap
- 2 tablespoons Argiletz white clay
- 5 drops Lavender essential oil
- 5 drops Lemon essential oil
-

Recipe:

Take a bowl and add cocoa butter, shea butter, coconut oil, almond oil and lemon juice. Take a deep pan and add water into it. Put that pan on the fire and heat it till it's got to 60 C. put that bowl over the pan having water. You need to be very careful that the bowl does not touch the pan directly. Grate the castile soap and add it to the bowl. Now blend all these mixtures with the help of stick blender. When a smooth mixture is formed, take it off the flame. Allow it to cool a little bit. Now pour them into jars and allow setting for a week. Your body wash is ready to be used.

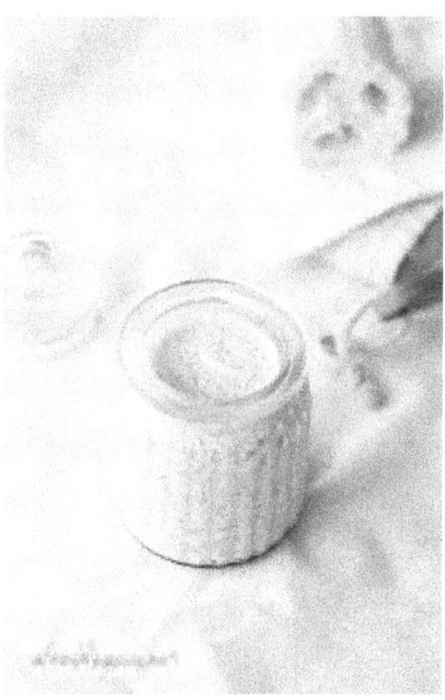

Grapefruit Body Mist

Ingredients:

- vodka

- distilled water

- 15 drops of grapefruit essential oil

- dark-glass spray bottle

Directions:

Fill a spray bottle two-thirds with vodka and add in essential oil then top with distilled water and shake before you use.

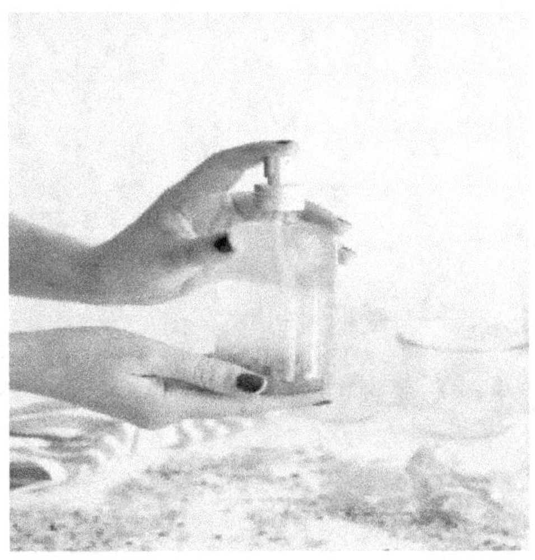

Dandelion Salve Recipe

Ingredients:

- one bowl of dried dandelions
- one cup of grapeseed oil
- twelve drops of lavender essential oil
- one quarter of a cup of beeswax

Directions:

In a double broiler boil the dandelions and oil over simmer. Heat for about three hours on simmer. Then use a cheesecloth to stress the oil and collect it in container, discard the dandelions.

Put the oil back into the heat-proof bowl in double broiler and add in beeswax, heat over medium heat until the beeswax has melted, remove from heat and stir. Add in your essential oil and mix well. Store in a glass jar with secure lid and keep in the fridge up to two months.

Oatmeal and lavender body wash:

This body wash made out of lavender and oatmeal is will soften your body skin and will also control oil.

Ingredients:

- 3 cups of water
- ¼ cup oatmeal
- ¼ cup castile soap
- 1 teaspoon vitamin E oil
- 2 teaspoon jojoba oil
- 10 drops of lavender essential oil

Recipe:

Take the bar of Castile soap and grate it in small pieces. Take a pan and put 3 cups of water into it. Bring this water to boil. Take a bowl and put oatmeal into it. Now transfer half of the water to oatmeal and half of it to castile soap. Keep on mixing water with castile soap. Leave water in the oatmeal for almost 1 hour. Strain this water and discard the oatmeal. Now add this filtered water to the castile soap. Add oils to the mixture and mix it well till a smooth mixture is formed. Your Oatmeal and lavender body wash are ready to use.

Cardamom & Vanilla Mist

Ingredients:

- half a cup of distilled water
- one teaspoon of vanilla extract
- six cardamom seeds

Directions:

Crack the cardamom seeds to reveal their pods. Add bits of cardamom to a saucepan with water and bring to a boil.

Remove this from heat. Allow the cardamom water to cool completely. Add scented water to a spray bottle. Add in the vanilla then shake well before using. Store bottle in cool and dry place.

Capsaicin Pain Relief Salve

Ingredients:

- one cup of grapeseed oil
- one quarter of a cup of beeswax
- three tablespoons of cayenne powder

Directions:

Add cayenne pepper, grapeseed oil, to a double broiler over medium heat then add in beeswax. Heat over medium heat until the beeswax is melted. Remove from heat and then put in the fridge and chill for ten minutes. Remove from fridge and whisk then add to glass jar with secure lid. This should keep for two months if you keep in the fridge.

Clay bodies wash:

This body wash with clay as its main ingredient will allow you to absorb extra oil from your body. Clay also has scrubbing properties that will also remove dead skin from your body making it fresh. With the addition of essential oil, it will also add smoothness and shine to your body.

Ingredients:

- 1 cup Castile liquid soap
- 1 tablespoon clay
- 3 tablespoon honey
- 2 teaspoon oil (jojoba, sweet almond, grape seed, sesame, or olive)
- 1 teaspoon vitamin E oil
- 2 teaspoon of essential oil (Chamomile, Geranium, Grapefruit, Lavender, Rosemary or Tea tree)

Recipe:

Take a blender and all the ingredients together. Blend them till a smooth mixture is formed. Store it in a beautiful glass jar for use.

When you go to take a bath, Take a small amount of this on the wash cloth and rub it over wet skin. Make a good amount of lather and rinse it off with the help of water.

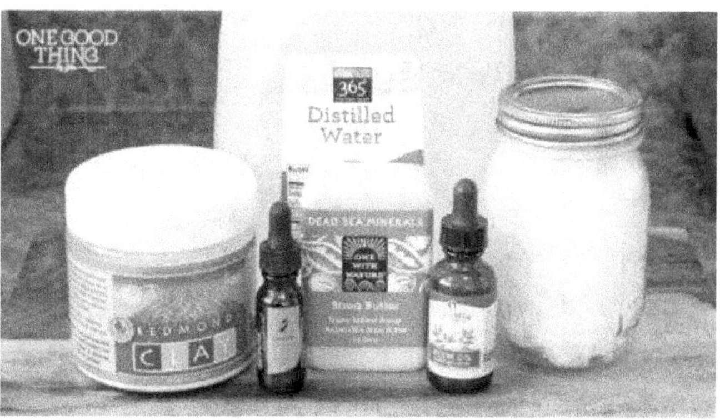

Tropical Homemade Body Mist

Ingredients:

- six teaspoons of grapefruit essential oil drops
- 20 Neroli essential oil drops
- one and a half tablespoons of coconut oil

- one and a half tablespoons of vegetable glycerin

- one and a half teaspoons of vodka

- two teaspoons of vanilla extract

- 10ml of Rose Hydrosol

- one and a half ounces of distilled water

Directions:

Fill up a spray bottle with Rose Hydrosol and water. Add in the vegetable glycerin, add in the coconut oil. Mix well. Add in the essential oils close and shake well. Let is rest for a few hours then shake it again before use.

Extra-Strength Pain Relief Salve

Ingredients:

- one quarter of a cup of beeswax

- three cups of grapeseed oil

- four tablespoons of Habanero powder

Directions:

Add in Habanero powder to a double broiler along with grapeseed oil over medium hea then add in the beeswax and stir leave on until the beeswax is melted. Remove from heat and put in the fridge for ten minutes. Remove and whisk then put in glass jar and seal with lid and place back in your fridge for up to two months.

Neem body wash:

This body wash is all set to go for oily skin. All you need to gather the stuff and prepare it at your home. The neem leaf that has also been added help to fight bacteria and it als has oil controlling properties. The addition of oil will give you silky smooth skin.

Ingredient:

- 6 cups distilled water
- ½ bar of shea butter soap
- ½ cup coconut oil
- 1 tablespoon clay
- Neem leaf extract
- Essential Oil (Chamomile, Geranium, Grapefruit, Lavender, Rosemary or Tea tree)

Recipe:

Start to chop shea butter bar into a form of powder. Take a stainless steel pan and add water into it. Bring this water to boil and now add shea butter soap powder into it. Cook it till a smooth mixture is formed. As the soap is melted, add coconut oil into it. Take clay in a bowl and add water into it so a thick paste is formed. Now add this paste of the clay in the pot having shea butter. As all the mixture is turned into a smooth blend, take it off the flame and put it into the containers to let it cool. As it dries, again mix all of the things with the help of a whisk. Now add neem extract and 10 drops of essential oil of your choice into it. Your neem body wash is ready to be used.

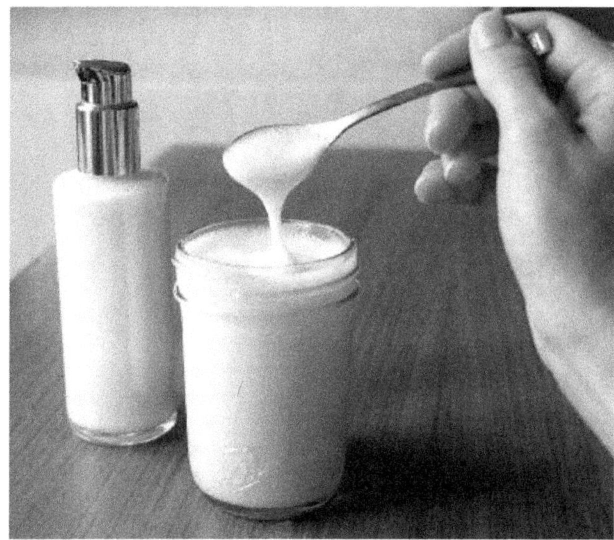

Aloe & Cucumber Body Mist

Ingredients:

- one cucumber

- one and a half teaspoons of Aloe Vera Gel

- juice from one lemon

- one tablespoon of Rosewater

- distilled water

Directions:

Peel the cucumber and dice it up into little pieces. Place into blender and pulse on high for a minute or so. Cover the bowl with some cheesecloth and then strain the cucumber juice into the bowl.

Add juice to spray bottle. Add the rest of the ingredients and shake well. Store mix in the fridge so it doesn't spoil. It will last about one week.

Cinnamon & Turmeric Pain Reducer Salve

Ingredients:

- three cups of grapeseed oil

- four tablespoons of turmeric

- one quarter of a cup of beeswax

- four tablespoons of cinnamon, ground

- four tablespoons of cayenne, ground

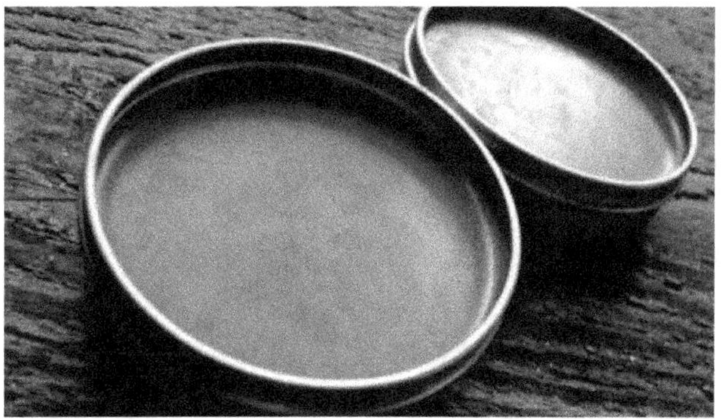

Directions:

Mix in a bowl cinnamon, turmeric, and cayenne. In a double broiler add in grapeseed oil and cinnamon mix and stir until well-blended. Heat over medium heat then add in beeswax and stir and cook until the beeswax is melted then remove from heat.

Put in the fridge to chill for ten minutes. Remove from fridge and whisk. Add to glass jar and place back into the fridge. This is a great salve that will help improve your circulation, and will help get the vitamins your bones need as they will deliver oxygen to your bones. This is good to use especially if you suffer from osteoarthritis.

Rosemary body wash

This rosemary body wash has all the essential ingredients that are necessary for your body. Citric acid has been added that will increase the shelf life of the body wash and it is also antibacterial.

Ingredients:

- 1 tablespoon oats
- 1 tablespoon of rosemary
- 1 cup of distilled water
- 1 teaspoon citric acid

- 2 tablespoon coconut oil (you can also use olive, grape seed, almond, jojoba, apricot kernel or any other oil)
- 1 tablespoon honey
- 1-1/2 cup liquid castile soap
- I teaspoon guar gum
- 30 drops essential oils (lavender, chamomile or lemongrass)

Recipe:

Take a kettle and add water into it. Bring this water to boil. Now, add oats and rosemary to the water. Cook them for 5 minutes. Remove it from the heat and cover it with a lid. Keep this for 15 minutes. Now, strain his infusion and discard rosemary and oats. Take bowl and add honey, oil, and citric acid together. Mix hem with the help of a whisk. Now start adding this infusion. Now add castile soap into it and mix it. Start sprinkling guar gum and keep on mixing with the whisk as the guar gum can get thickened and form a clump. Now add your optional essential oil into it. Transfer all these in a bottle from where you can use it. Your rosemary body wash is ready to use.

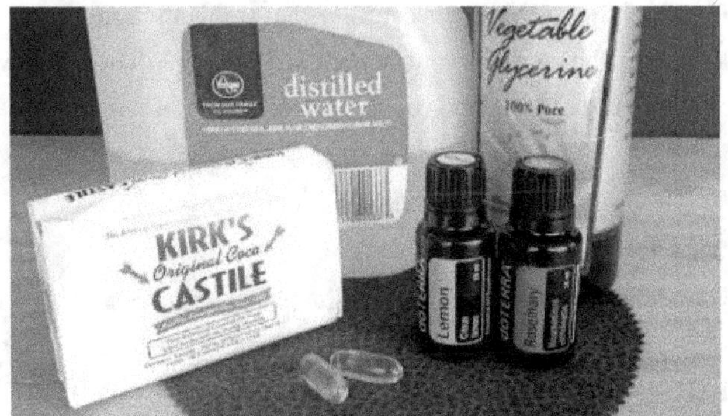

Forest Scent Body Mist

Ingredients:

- three drops of fir needle essential oil

- three drops of cedarwood essential oil

- five drops of spruce essential oil

- five drops of Bergamot essential oil

- five drops of Vetiver essential oil

- one teaspoon of Jojoba oil

- distilled water

Directions:

In a spray bottle add in your jojoba oil and essential oils along with some distilled water. Shake well before using.

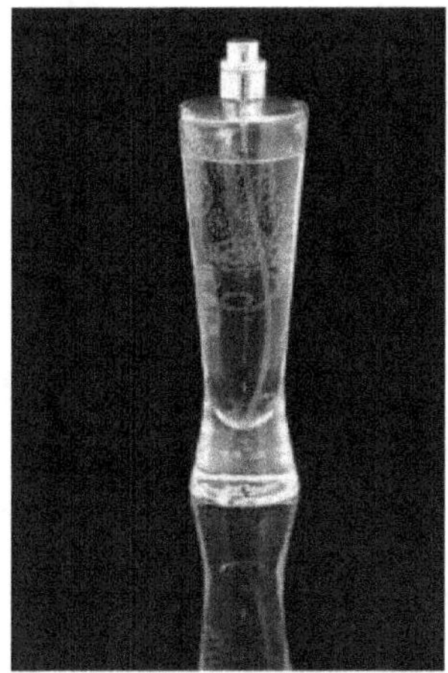

Salve for Aching & Sore Muscles

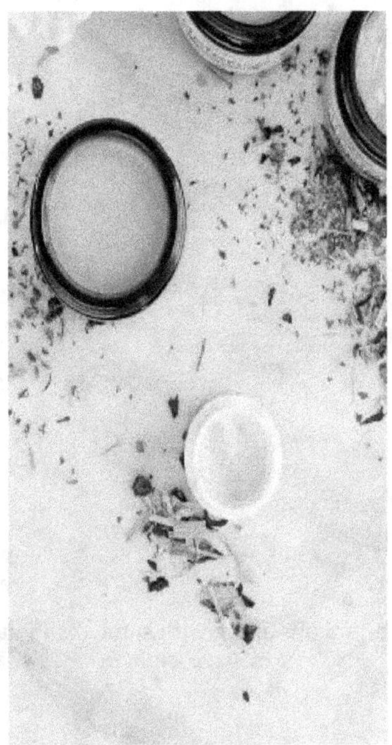

Ingredients:

- two tablespoons of beeswax

- one quarter of a cup of almond oil

- one quarter of a cup of coconut oil

- one quarter of a teaspoon of cinnamon, ground

- one quarter of a teaspoon of black pepper, freshly ground

- 25 drops of peppermint essential oil

- 20 drops of eucalyptus essential oil

- 20 drops of clove oil

Directions:

In a double broiler in a heat-proof bowl add your base oils—almond oil and coconut oil. Add in cinnamon and black pepper. Bring water to a boil then reduce to simmer. Remove from heat after 20 minutes and allow to steep.

Allow to steep for an hour and then re-heat adding beeswax over medium heat. Heat and stir until the beeswax has melted. Remove from heat then add in the essential oils and mix well. Let sit at room temperature for three hours then apply this salve onto your sore muscles directly.

Glycerin body wash

This is a sort of basic body wash that can go perfectly with normal skin type. You can use it with great ease. The glycerin has been added that will give smoothness to your skin.

Ingredients:

- 4 cups distilled water
- 1 bar Castile soap
- 2 tablespoons Glycerin
- 2 vial or 2 tablespoons of Vitamin E
- 20 drops essential oils of your choice (Chamomile, Geranium, Grapefruit, Lavender, Rosemary or Tea tree)

Recipe:

Grate the castile soap bar into the form of powder. Take a stainless steel pan and add water into it. Heat it till it gets a boil. Turn the heat low and start adding powdered castile soap into it. Keep on mixing this with the help of a whisk. When all the castile soap is mixed with water, remove it from heat. Now add essential oil, vitamin E and glycerin into it. Allow it to cool and let it set for 24 hours. After 24 hours, again mix all the ingredients. Transfer it to the glass bottle or container of your choice. Your Glycerin body wash is ready for use.

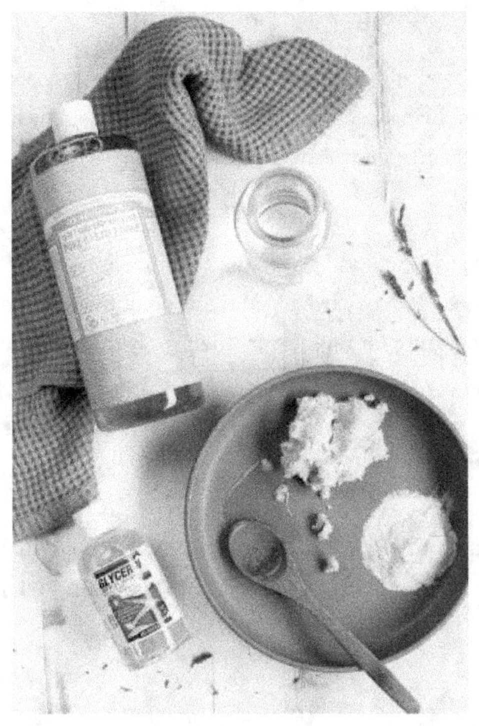

Vanilla, Lemon & Lavender Body Spray

Ingredients:

- three and a half ounces of witch hazel

- six drops of lemon essential oil

- 35 drops of vanilla essential oil

- 20 drops of Lavender essential oil

Directions:

Add all of your ingredients into a glass spray bottle. Make sure to shake well before every use.

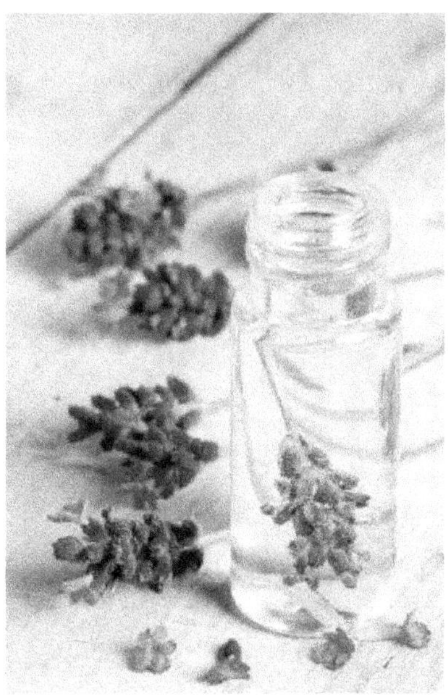

Herbal Salve

Ingredients:

- one quarter cup of almond oil

- one quarter cup of coconut oil

- one quarter cup of beeswax

- eight drops of grapefruit essential oil

- ten drops of rose essential oil

- ten drops of peppermint essential oil

Directions:

In a small pot heat your base oils and beeswax over medium heat until the beeswax has melted. Remove from heat and add in the essential oils and mix well. Then add to glass jar with secure lid.

Aloe Vera body wash

Aloe Vera has been used for its medicinal and beauty care properties. It has nurturing and soothing properties that make it distinct from other things. This Aloe Vera body wash is the product of choice for normal skin.

Ingredients:

- 1 cup aloe Vera gel
- 1 cup castile soap
- 2 tablespoon glycerin
- 1 cup water
- 10 drops of essential oil (Chamomile, Geranium, Grapefruit, Lavender, Rosemary or Tea tree)

Recipe:

Take a pan and add water into it. Bring this water to boil. Start adding castile soap and mix it well. Take it off the heat. Take half an aloe Vera and peel it. Take out its pulp that should make roughly 1 cup. Put that pulp into the blender and blend it till a smooth mixture is formed. Add this pulp to castile soap and mix it well. Now add glycerin and essential oil to the mixture and mix them. Allow it to cool and set for 12 hours. Mix it again with the help of a whisk. Transfer it to clean containers. Your Aloe Vera body wash is ready to use.

Moisturizing Body Mist

Ingredients:

- one and a half teaspoons of grapeseed oil

- six drops of vitamin E oil

- two teaspoons of vegetable glycerin

- 20 drops of vanilla essential oil

- one tablespoon of witch hazel

- distilled water

Directions:

Add all of your ingredients into a glass spray bottle and shake well before each use. Great to use just after a shower, rub it into your skin.

Purifying Body Mist

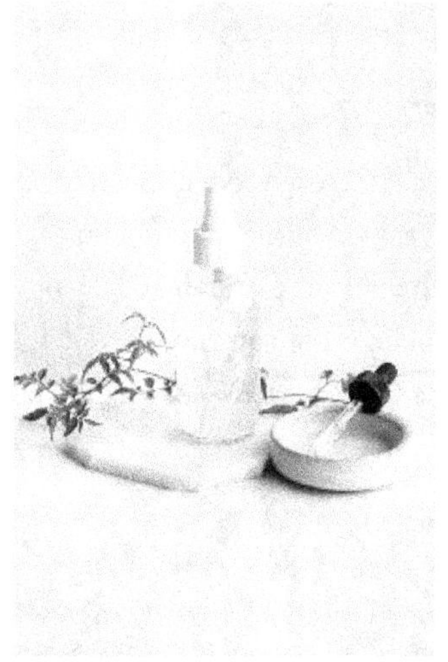

Ingredients:

- 40 drops of eucalyptus essential oil

- 35 drops of lemon essential oil

- 25 drops of peppermint essential oil

- distilled water

- two tablespoons of witch hazel

Directions:

Add ingredients into dark glass spray bottle and shake well before each use.

Raw Honey & Aloe Vera Burn Salve

Ingredients:

- three tablespoons of coconut oil

- one quarter of a cup of raw honey

- three tablespoons of aloe vera

Directions:

Mix your ingredients in a small pot over medium heat, use a wooden spoon to mix. Remove from heat and add to glass jar. Clean the area of burned skin first using some apple cider vinegar. Using this treatment can help to recover vitamins to the burned skin and will help restore the pH balance of your skin. After you have applied the salve cover it with gauze. Do not use this treatment on serious burns—seek medical attention

Vanilla & Orange Natural Body Mist

Ingredients:

- 20 drops of orange essential oil
- one teaspoon of vanilla extract
- half an ounce of vegetable glycerin
- half an ounce of witch hazel
- distilled water

Directions:

Shake all ingredients in a small glass spray bottle. Make sure to shake well before each use.

Burst of Citrus Energy Body Mist

Ingredients:

- half an ounce of witch hazel
- half an ounce of vegetable glycerin
- 20 drops of grapefruit essential oil
- six drops of lime essential oil
- six drops of lemon essential oil
- distilled water

Directions:

Mix all of your ingredients in a small glass spray bottle make sure to shake well before each use.

Lavender & Chamomile Hand Salve

Ingredients:

- one quarter of a cup of beeswax

- one quarter of a cup of almond oil

- one quarter of a cup of coconut oil

- one quarter of a cup of lavender, dried

- one quarter of a cup of chamomile, dried

- ten drops of lavender essential oil

- five drops of Eucalyptus essential oil

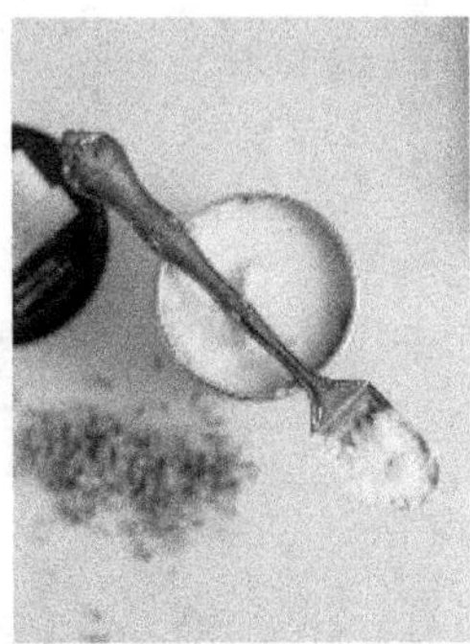

Directions:

In a saucepan over medium heat add in your almond oil, coconut oil, lavender, and chamomile. Stir until it becomes hot. Lower heat to simmer and continue to cook for another hour.

Remove from heat then stress the oil through a cheesecloth and discard the herbs. Add the oil back into saucepan along with beeswax over medium heat until the beeswax has melted. Remove from heat and add in essential oils, mix well. Add to glass jar first allow it to cool for a bit. Seal jar with a secure lid.

Orange Blossom Body Mist

Ingredients:

- 40 drops of orange essential oil
- one teaspoon of vegetable glycerin
- half an ounce of witch hazel
- distilled water

Directions:

Add ingredients into glass spray bottle and shake well. Shake before each use and when using it rub into skin.

Chickweed Oil & Comfrey Salve

Ingredients:

- half a cup of chickweed oil
- two ounces of comfrey, dried leaves
- twenty drops of lavender essential oil
- one quarter cup of beeswax

Directions:

In a double broiler add the chickweed oil and the comfrey leaves bring to a boil. Reduce to simmer and continue to cook for another hour. Remove from heat and then stress the oil through cheesecloth, discard herbs.

Add the oil back into double broiler along with beeswax over medium heat. Heat until the beeswax is melted, then remove from heat add in the essential oil and mix well. Add to glass jar with secure lid and keep in the fridge.

Patchouli Body Spray

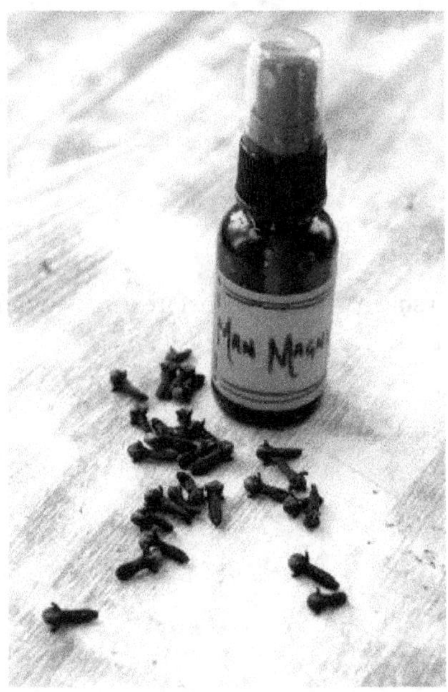

Ingredients:

- half a teaspoon of Tunisian Patchouli essential oil

- half an ounce of vegetable glycerin

- half an ounce of witch hazel

- distilled water

Directions:

Mix all ingredients in small glass spray bottle and shake well before each use.

Healing Salve

Ingredients:

- one cup of coconut oil

- one cup of almond oil

- two ounces of comfrey leaf, dried

- three tablespoons of plantain leaf, dried

- one teaspoon of echinacea root

- one quarter of a cup of beeswax

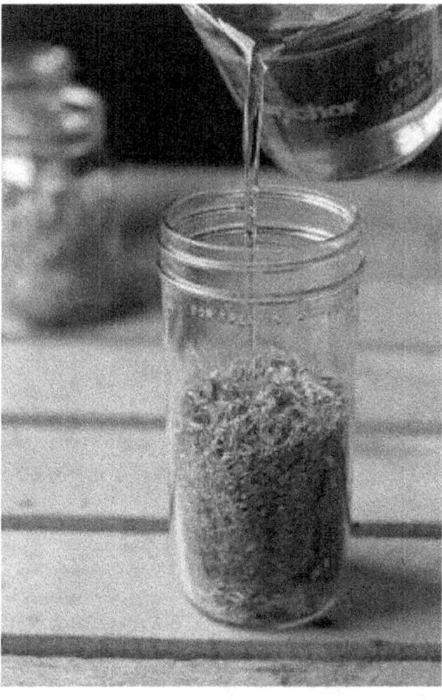

Directions:

Add your herbs to your base oils in a double broiler and bring to a boil then reduce to a simmer for one hour. Remove from heat then stress the oil through cheesecloth.

Discard the herbs and put the oil back into the double broiler along with the beeswax over medium heat. Heat until the beeswax has melted and remove from heat. Add in the echinacea root and mix well. Add to small tins for storing. Use this salve on poison ivy, diaper rash, or other injuries of the skin.

Vanilla Coffee Body Mist

Ingredients:

- six coffee essential oil drops

- 20 vanilla oleoresin drops

- half an ounce of witch hazel

- distilled water

Directions:

Mix all ingredients in dark glass spray bottle. Shake well before each application.

Vapor Rub

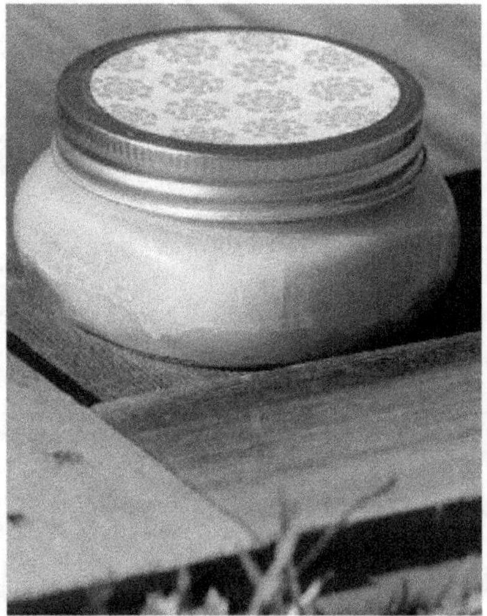

Ingredients:

- half a cup of almond oil

- one quarter of a cup of beeswax

- twelve drops of cinnamon essential oil

- twelve drops of rosemary essential oil

- twenty drops of eucalyptus essential oil

- twenty drops of peppermint essential oil

Directions:

In a double broiler add in the almond oil and the beeswax over medium heat. Heat until the wax has melted and stir. Remove from heat and add in the essential oils and mix well. Put into small storing tins. This can be used on chest to help ease congestion and coughing.

Sweet Orange & Vanilla Body Mist

Ingredients:

- 20 vanilla oleoresin drops

- 20 sweet orange essential oil drops

- half an ounce of witch hazel

- distilled water

Directions:

Add all of your ingredients into small dark-glass spray bottle and make sure to shake before each use.

Comfort & Soothing Salve

Ingredients:

- half a cup of grapeseed oil

- half a cup of coconut oil

- half a tablespoon of vitamin E oil

- one quarter of a cup of beeswax

- eight drops of Rose, Melaleuca, Cypress, Frankincense and Eucalyptus essential oils

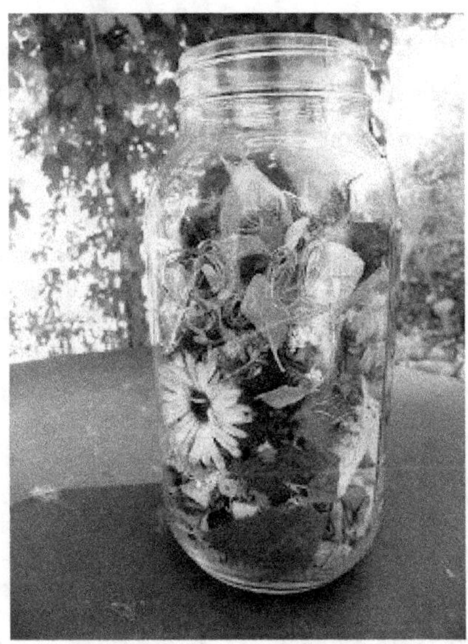

Directions:

In a double broiler add in the base oils—grapeseed and coconut along with the beeswax over medium heat. Cook until the beeswax is melted stirring occasionally. Remove from heat and add in the vitamin E oil and essential oils, mix well. Add to jars and allow to set for a couple of hours before use. Apply this salve to skin or chest area.

Ylang-Ylang & Vanilla Body Mist

Ingredients:

- 20 vanilla oleoresin drops

- four Ylang-Ylang essential oil drops

- half an ounce of witch hazel

- distilled water

Directions:

Add all of your ingredients into a dark-glass spray bottle make sure to shake well before each use.

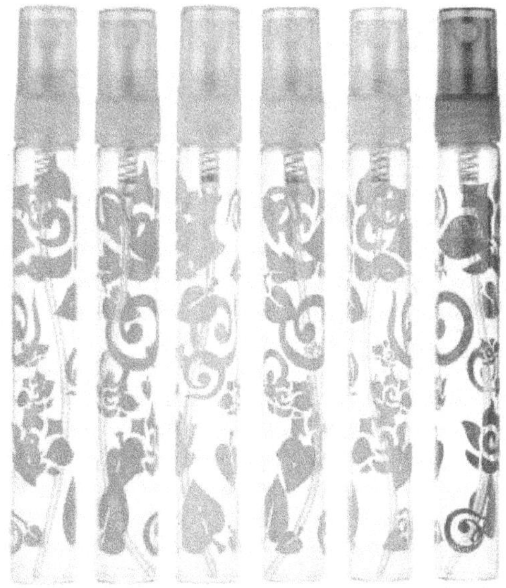

Tea Tree Body Mist

Ingredients:

- 25 drops of tea tree essential oil

- half an ounce of witch hazel

- distilled water

Directions:

Add your ingredients into a dark-glass spray bottle and shake well before each use.

Marigold & Vanilla Body Mist

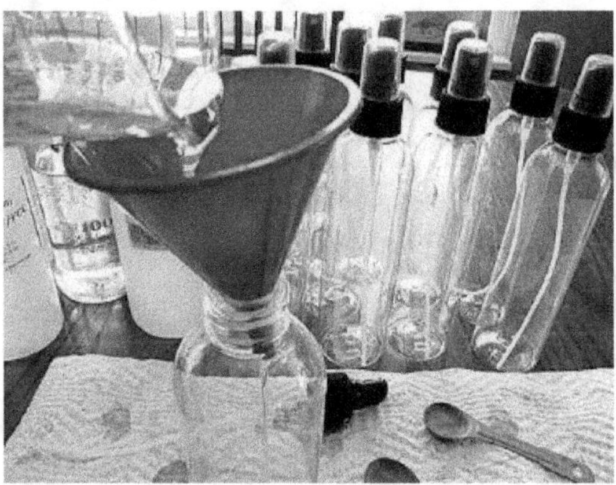

Ingredients:

- 30 drops of marigold essential oil

- 20 drops of vanilla oleoresin

- half an ounce of witch hazel

- distilled water

Directions:

Add all of your ingredients into dark-glass spray bottle shake well before each and every use. The scent of marigold in this spray will help to keep the pesky bugs at bay.

Latenight Perfume

Ingredients:

- six tablespoons of witch hazel

- three tablespoons of Jojoba oil

- two and a half tablespoons of distilled water

- 10 drops of lavender essential oil

- 15 drops of clove essential oil

- 8 drops of cedarwood essential oil

Materials needed:

- coffee filter

- funnel

- two dark-glass spray bottles

Directions:

Clean the bottles out with some hot soapy water. You can also put them in your dishwasher to sterilize them. Add a lid to one of them and set it aside.

Add your carrier oil into one of the bottles. Add in essential oils. Add in witch hazel. Add lid to this bottle and shake well. Allow this bottle to rest for forty-eight hours to a couple of weeks.

The scent will be at its strongest at about six weeks. Check it weekly and once you get the scent you want add two tablespoons of distilled water and shake for a minute or so. Put the coffee filter into the funnel.

Transfer the liquid from the bottle it is in to a nice perfume bottle. Label it and store it in a cool and dark place.

Lavender Citrus Homemade Perfume

Ingredients:

- 15 drops of Bergamot essential oil
- 15 drops of lavender essential oil
- 12 drops of lemon essential oil
- 12 drops of sweet orange essential oil
- two teaspoons of beeswax
- two teaspoons of Jojoba oil

Directions:

Add your Jojoba oil and beeswax in a pan heat over medium heat until beeswax is melted. Remove from heat and add in essential oils mix well. Then add mix to small tin and allow to harden. Cover with lid.

Sweet Citrus Sunshine Homemade Perfume

Ingredients:

- 10 drops of grapefruit essential oil

- 10 drops of sweet orange essential oil

- 10 drops of peppermint essential oil

- two tablespoons of witch hazel

- one tablespoon of Jojoba oil

- 10 drops of lavender oil

- distilled water

Directions:

Add jojoba oil to glass container then add in the witch hazel. Add in the essential oils and mix. Add in distilled water.

Transfer to a dark-glass container for up to six weeks. The longer you leave it to sit the stronger the scent will be. After you have reached the scent that you desire transfer into a nice attractive spray bottle.

Chapter 3 Essential Oils for Treating Stress and Anxiety

There are three different methods through which you can use essential oils to relieve stress and anxiety:

Topical Application:

It is the process of placing the essential oil on your nails, teeth, mouth, hair, skin or mucous membrane of the body. The oils penetrate into the skin rapidly when they touch it directly.

It is important to blend and dilute the essential oils in a carrier substance. Carrie materials include coconut, avocado, olive, jojoba, and sweet almond oil. You can apply this blend on rims of your ears, bottoms of your feet, or directly to the affected area. You can also take them through massage, in baths, and by compresses.

Oral Application:

You can also ingest essential oils through the mouth. It is critical to consult a professional to determine if the ingesting oils are pure and safe. They mix many essential oils with synthetics which is not healthy.

The most efficient manner of ingesting essential oils is by mixing one drop of any oil of your preference in one teaspoon of honey or a glass of water. You can also add a few drops (maximum three) of the chosen essential oil underneath your tongue. It is an effective method because capillaries are present closely to the surface of tissue underneath your tongue and thus, the healing components of th oils transfer to the bloodstream rapidly.

You can also take essential oils orally through other options such as cooking, making tea, adding two to three drops to beverages, and capsules.

Aromatherapy:

It is very popular. Our sense of smell can trigger powerful emotional responses. Molecules of the essential oils enter into the nasal cavity. It stimulates the limbic system of the brain. Resultantly, the calming responses such as blood pressure, production of hormones, breathing patterns, and heart rate regulate the stress.

There are many ways to take aromatherapy such as through diffusers, cologne, perfume, vent, fan, humidifier or vaporizer, as direct inhalation, hot water vapor, and in a bath. It is best for relieving tension.

Top Essential Oils Blends for Stress and Anxiety:

Essential oils elicit emotional reactions. They uplift your emotions and thus, proven to be suitable for treating depression, stress, and anxiety. Here are some of the best essential oils blends to relieve stress and anxiety:

Frankincense Essential Oil:

It provides a peaceful and calming energy. It also provides spiritual grounding. It quiets the mind and deepens the meditation. You can mix it with lavender and bergamot oils in 1:1 ratio to make the massage oil for hands. It has a positive effect on depression and pain.

It is ideal for spiritual enlightenment. Diffuse a few drops of this essential oil using your diffuser while reading, meditating or praying. It increases spiritual awareness.

Lavender Essential Oil:

It is the most versatile and popular essential oil. It is ideal for combating stress, and anxiety. It is helpful in providing relaxation and heart health. It reduces, according to a study, serum cortisol. This hormone plays a critical role in the way your body responding to stress and developing a healthy cardiovascular system.

You can make a detox bath for relieving anxiety by mixing lavender oil with sea salt and Epsom salts to a warm water bath. It rejuvenates your body.

Add a few drops of lavender and cedarwood essential oil in any unscented lotion. Massaging this cream on your skin rejuvenates your spiritual health.

To relieve tension, add a few drops (maximum three) of lavender essential oil on your palms, massage it on your hands and smell it.

Sweet Orange Essential Oil:

All citrus essential oils are high in uplifting the energy levels and boosting the moods. A study found that providing smaller doses of sweet orange essential oil to patients with depression is effective in combating the situation.

It is also useful in alleviating insomnia. Spray a few drops of sweet orange oil mixed wit lavender oil on your pillow before going to bed.

Bergamot Essential Oil:

It is a part of the citrus family. Ten minutes of weekly inhalation of this essential oil has shown a significantly positive effect in combating anxiety, balancing nerves, reducing heart rate, and blood pressure.

Make a mix of peppermint, grapefruit, and bergamot essential oil in equal concentration. Combine it with any carrier substance. Inhaling it during the day increases your strength and helps you to alleviate stress and anxiety.

Chamomile Essential Oil:

It contains a peaceful, calming scent. It decreases worry, anxiety, over-thinking, and irritability and enhances inner harmony. It is safe to use.

For immediate relaxation, apply a few drops (maximum four) of each peppermint, lavender, and chamomile essential oil on your temples. It provides a cooling effect.

Jasmine Essential Oil:

It is an amazing essential oil for relieving anxiety. You can wear it as a natural perfume. Simple rub two to three drops of jasmine essential oil on your wrist. You can also use lavender and vanilla essential oils in the same manner if you are a woman. For men, clove and cypress oils are the best options.

Chapter 4 Aromatherapy for Weight Loss

Weight Loss with Essential Oils:

Many essential oils play an active role in helping you shed the unwanted fats.

Fennel Essential Oil:

Fennel essential oil is a source of melatonin. It is the natural hormone that regulates wake-sleep cycles. It creates beige fat instead of white fat in your body and helps you achieve your weight loss goals. Beige fat burns off as energy whereas the later is stored for energy.

Fennel oil also suppresses appetite and improves digestion. So, the fennel seeds are consumed in the fasting days to reduce hunger. Scientists carried out an experiment on rats. The mice inhaled fennel oil for ten minutes twice a day. Resultantly, they showed a faster rate of digestion and consumed lesser calories as well.

Bergamot Essential Oil:

Depression and anxiety can lead to emotional eating in some people. They get a temporary sense of relief and comfort in it. But it has its long-term adverse effects such as the feelings of self-criticism and guilt.

Scientists have discovered that aromatherapy with bergamot essential oil can break this vicious cycle. Just fifteen minutes of inhaling bergamot oil results in increased energy and improved positive emotions. The scientists also tested saliva for cortisol. It is a hormone that is released as a response by the body to stress. They found that people inhaling bergamot oil had the lesser quantity of cortisol in their saliva than the ones who did not inhale it.

Cinnamon Essential Oil:

Insulin metabolizes fats and carbohydrates in our bodies by facilitating the absorption of blood sugar by either storing it as fat or converting it to energy. Insulin resistance occurs in the body when cells stop responding to insulin. The body starts storing fat instead of burning it. Resultantly, the person does not only gain weight but also find difficulty in losing it. It is a precursor for Type 2 Diabetes. Cinnamon essential oil has shown to help to increase the rate of blood sugar glucose uptake by heightening the insulin sensitivity in the body.

Metabolism syndrome is a confluence of disorders such as high blood cholesterol, high blood sugar, high blood pressure, insulin resistance, abdominal obesity, and impaired glucose tolerance. Up to 25% of Americans suffer from it. Certain inflammatory cells are also found responsible for obesity in the human body. Aromatherapy with cinnamon essential oil inhibits production of these cells in our bodies. It is a fundamental element in the journey of losing weight.

Peppermint Essential Oil:

Peppermint has many medicinal benefits. It contains 70% menthol. It treats indigestion. It is also an effective muscle relaxer. When used with caraway essential oil, peppermint extracts improve the flow of bile, reduce bloating, and ease the muscles of the stomach.

Researchers have found that pitting peppermint against ylang-ylang and inhaling in the peppermint aromatherapy results in calmer moods, improved memory function, and better alertness. It is also an effective natural appetite suppressor. Volunteers inhaled peppermint essential oil every two hours and reported in consuming significantly fewer calories and lower hunger levels.

Lemon Essential Oil:

Lemon contains limonene which has incredible fat-dissolving powers. Researchers found that combining lemon and grapefruits extracts increased lipolysis.

Lemon essential oil is a powerful mood booster and mainly alleviates negative feelings. It also raises the levels of a neurotransmitter and stress hormone norepinephrine. It is responsible for fight-or-flight mechanism. It increases the level of oxygen in the brain. It improves cognitive function. It also ramps up blood flow and heart rate which results in muscles working better and faster. It is also a great pain reliever. It soothes down strained muscles and aches.

Homemade Aromatic Essential Oil Blends:

You can blend essential oils to get your favorite scents along with achieving the high quality of healing powers of the oils. Some of the tried-and-true blends of essential oils for losing weight are:

Craving Curbing Slave:

Combine twenty-four drops of patchouli, forty drops of bergamot, and eighty drops of fennel oil with half cup of olive oil. Massage this mix on your abdomen.

Metabolism Boosting Soak:

Add eight drops of grapefruit, ten drops of cypress, ten drops of rosemary, and two tablespoons of jojoba oil in the bath water. Soak in it for twenty to thirty minutes.

Appetite Suppressing Diffusion:

Combine twelve drops of peppermint, twelve drops of ginger, twenty drops of lemon, and forty drops of mandarin oil. Add a few drops of this mix in your diffuser and inhale

Rejuvenating Bath:

Add lemon, sandalwood, orange, ginger, and grapefruit essential oils (maximum five drops each) in your bath water.

Anti-Cellulite Rub:

Combine two drops of ginger, two drops of peppermint, two drops of cypress, five drops of rosemary, and ten drops of grapefruit essential oil. Blend them with any carrier substance. Apply on your skin.

Fat Reducing Massage:

Combine five drops each of cypress, lemon, and grapefruit essential oil with a quarter cup of almond oil. Massage the mix on your body.